Collaborative Care
Nursing Case Management

Mary Lou Salome Etheredge, R.N., M.S.
Editor

The Center for Nursing Case Management
New England Medical Center Hospitals

American Hospital Publishing, Inc.,
a wholly owned subsidiary
of the American Hospital Association

Library of Congress Catalog-in-Publication Data
Collaborative care : nursing case management / Mary Lou Salome Etheredge.
   p.   cm.
ISBN 1-55648-032-6
1. Primary nursing—Administration. I. Etheredge, Mary Lou Salome.
RT90.7.C65   1989   89–281
362.1'73'068—dc19   CIP

Catalog no. 154151

©1989 by American Hospital Publishing, Inc.,
a wholly owned subsidiary of the American Hospital Association

Text set in Trump
2.5M—4/89—0234
3M—6/90—0270
1M—6/93—0353

Audrey Kaufman, Project Editor
Linda Conheady, Manuscript Editor
Marcia Bottoms, Managing Editor
Peggy DuMais, Production Coordinator
Marcia Vecchione, Designer
Brian Schenk, Books Division Director

Contents

About the Editor

Mary Lou Salome Etheredge, R.N., M.S., is director of staff education at New England Medical Center Hospitals and director of programs and publications for The Center for Nursing Case Management. She has published and lectures nationally on management development, managed care and case management, and early childhood development issues for parents and child care providers.

List of Figures

List of Tables

Contributors

Kathleen A. Bower, R.N., M.S.N., director of research and development, The Center for Nursing Case Management

Ann Downey-Dezell, R.N., B.S.N., project director for patient acuity, New England Medical Center Hospitals

Paul Drew, vice-president, clinical operations, medicine, New England Medical Center Hospitals

Jacqueline Gannon-Somerville, R.N., M.S.N., nurse manager, New England Medical Center Hospitals

Jerome H. Grossman, M.D., president, New England Medical Center Hospitals

Kenneth Miller, M.D., chief, leukemia services, New England Medical Center Hospitals, and assistant professor of medicine, Tufts University School of Medicine

Cheryl B. Stetler, R.N., Ph.D., former special assistant for nursing research, New England Medical Center Hospitals

Sandra Twyon, R.N., M.S.N., chairman, department of nursing, New England Medical Center Hospitals, and chief executive officer, The Center for Nursing Case Management

Peter Van Etten, executive vice-president and chief financial officer, New England Medical Center Hospitals

Karyl Woldum, R.N., M.S.N., vice-chairman, medicine, department of nursing, New England Medical Center Hospitals

Karen Zander, R.N., M.S., C.S., organizational development specialist, New England Medical Center Hospitals, and director of consultation services, The Center for Nursing Case Management

Foreword

For generations, nurses have responded effectively to the environment in which it was necessary to deliver care. Florence Nightingale took on the ravages of war and the squalor of prison in the same spirit that we have taken on the prospective pricing system. Today, however, nurses are finding that the traditional dogmas of the past are inadequate to address the demanding issues of the present.

This book is significant because it provides a model for the timely, rational pursuit of acceptable contemporary health care outcomes. The professionals at The New England Medical Center Hospitals have responded to health care's driving force, distilling an evolutionary sequence into an outcome-driven model.

There have been times in nursing's history when nurses innovated at the expense of past achievements. Not this time! In designing the case management approach, the authors of this book have built on the success of primary nursing. A case manager is the primary nurse responsible for developing patient care outcomes for his or her caseload. Nurses, working closely with other professionals, manage services rendered during an episode of care in order to conserve funds and resources while ensuring the patient's right to acceptable outcomes.

In my years as a board member, and later as president, of the American Organization of Nursing Executives, I was privileged to meet hundreds of nurse executives, nurse managers, and primary nurses who affirmed the value of primary nursing to patients and their families, as well as to nurses and their patients' physicians. The continuity and accountability inherent in primary nursing, along with the bonding that takes place between patient and nurse, are important underpinnings of the case management model. For many of us, the accountability demanded by primary nursing implied addressing the outcomes of each step in the nursing process and, in many cases, the outcomes of the nursing care delivered. The case management model boldly takes on the complex mosaic of care for a patient during an entire episode. It addresses the outcome of the processes within that episodic mosaic—the targets met and not met.

Case management is a new way to provide clinically competent care to a patient; therefore, the need for more intensive education is critical for building new skills that will enhance our effectiveness as nurse/case managers. Built into this model is a rich but streamlined presentation that guides the nurse in the ways of case management, a natural extension of established nursing practice.

As we embark on this evolution of our practice—balancing the needs of our patients with our organizational obligations for efficiency in the health care system—let us keep clearly in mind our obligation to simultaneously manage the *caring* for our patient and his or her family. If nursing fails to guarantee the caring, it is unlikely that any other discipline will come forward to fill the void.

We can learn the cognitive skills necessary to become successful case managers. At the same time, we must retain that one precious core value from our traditional past—that is, we must manage the caring. Thus, as we grow in competence to meet contemporary health care demands, we use our individual strength for warmth, compassion, and humor, retaining the rewards of the spirit as we nurture those around us.

June Werner
Chairperson
Department of Nursing
The Evanston Hospital Corporation
Evanston, Illinois

Preface

Changes in health care, including the escalating number of acutely ill patients with shorter hospital stays, highlight the urgent need to rethink patient care needs and clinicians' roles. Nursing case management—the actual mobilization, monitoring, and rationalization of the resources that patients use over a course of illness—marks a new generation of technologies that offers the opportunity to objectively define quality care at the same time it revolutionizes nursing and integrates patient care activities.

The nursing case management model developed at New England Medical Center Hospitals evolved from a 13-year history of primary nursing after a 3-year investigation of nursing and physician practice patterns as they related to outcomes of care. Nursing case management as a professional practice model offers staff nurses substantial incentive by acknowledging their valuable and unique contributions as collaborating members of the health care team. The current nursing shortage only makes more cogent the need for this role redefinition. Although there has been an unprecedented surge in the number of strategies to entice nurses into the hospital setting, all fall short if they do not involve an in-depth examination of the staff nurse's role.

This patient-based approach is part of the heritage of New England Medical Center Hospitals. Founded in 1796 as the Boston Dispensary, New England Medical Center Hospitals is a highly specialized, 480-bed academic medical institution that has been dedicated to high-quality, compassionate patient care throughout its history.

A model as innovative as nursing case management would never have been conceived and could not have been developed without leaders with vision who met head-on the challenges of today's health care environment. This book is dedicated to those leaders.

Nursing Case Management: An Overview

The current and anticipated health care environment demands that nurses and other health care providers shift their focus from planned care to managed care. The emphasis on care planning has been a hallmark of nursing practice for decades, and it will continue to be an important component of nursing care. However, the need to ensure the achievement of acceptable patient outcomes within an effective time line and with an appropriate use of resources necessitates a reexamination of the processes for care. Comeau (1987) supports this by observing that

> . . . prospective payment has changed the health care product from a day of care (or a visit) to an entire case or episode of illness. More than just a new way of paying for care, it has changed our way of planning, managing, and thinking about health care.

Controlling health care costs is not the only challenge in today's practice environment. Consumers are becoming more emphatic about the need to maintain, or in some cases improve, the quality of care that is provided. They are concerned that costs may be reduced without regard to subsequent effects on quality. This suggests the need for a system of care delivery that will simultaneously reduce costs and ensure satisfactory patient outcomes. Case management addresses this two-part need. This care modality recognizes that an integral interrelationship exists among outcomes, cost, and process (figure 1-1, see p. 18) and that one factor cannot be altered without considering the effects on the other two.

This chapter will present an overview of the case management model—what it is; how it operates, particularly in relation to managed care; who the principal actors are and what kinds of skills and training they need; and how case management is viewed in the literature. It concludes with a rationale for the nurse as case manager. Successive chapters will expand on these themes. Case studies will be presented, and the impact of nursing case management on other areas of the institution will be described.

□ Case Management Defined

Case management is a system of patient care delivery that focuses on the achievement of outcomes within effective time frames and with appropriate use of resources. It encompasses an entire episode of illness, crossing all settings in which the patient receives care. Case management incorporates the principles of managed care as well as the principles of accountability for outcomes that come from primary nursing.

The focus of change in case management is the nurse's role because care is directed by a case manager who often is involved in a group practice, that is, a multiunit nursing group functioning in conjunction with key physicians. (The group practice model is further explained in chapter 2.) To increase their effectiveness, case managers usually focus on a specific patient population. Patient populations may be clustered by case type, by physician, or by a combination of the two. For example, case managers could manage the care of all patients within a given setting who are scheduled to have radical mastectomies. In other instances, case managers might manage the care of all patients who receive their medical care from a specific physician, or they might manage the care of all of Dr. X's leukemia patients.

The case manager is the primary nurse responsible for developing patient care outcomes for his or her caseload. The case manager is accountable for meeting outcomes within an appropriate length of stay, utilizing resources appropriately, and following established standards. The case manager is also responsible for collaborating with the health care team, the patient, and the patient's family to accomplish these outcomes.

Case managers have a unique role within nursing because their accountability is for the outcome of care (including length of stay and resource utilization) throughout an entire episode of illness. This distinguishes case management from other nursing care modalities in which accountability is limited to the outcomes within a given shift or unit.

☐ Managed Care: The Basis for Case Management

The essence of managed care is the organization of unit-based care so that specific patient outcomes can be achieved within fiscally responsible time frames (lengths of stay) while utilizing resources appropriate (in amount and sequence) to the specific case type and the individual patient. The term *unit* refers to the geographic area in which the patient receives care. Units may include areas such as inpatient or ambulatory units or the emergency department. Managed care can be implemented in any nursing care delivery system (for example, primary, team, or functional).

Managed care uses tools and systems to provide outcome-oriented, cost-effective care by taking existing information and making it more useful to practitioners. Specifically, managed care promotes the identification of expected outcomes, time frames, processes, and resources by case type before the patient's entry into the health care system. This allows clinicians to know in advance the outcomes they are working toward, how the outcomes will be attained, and the time frame in which they are working. Such knowledge increases the clinician's control of patient care. In addition, it strengthens interdisciplinary collaboration because each member of the team is clear about the expectations for time lines, care activities, and resource utilization.

Patient control and participation are also facilitated by knowledge of outcomes, time frames, and resource utilization because clinicians are able to share clearer expectations with patients and their families. Ultimately, this allows the patient more opportunity to plan his or her own care and anticipate its

3

outcome. For example, clinicians are generally aware of the usual length of stay and the discharge activity parameters for patients receiving care for a specific diagnosis. Often, however, the patient is not given specific information or is not given the information in a timely manner. The resulting confusion sets up a situation in which prolonged length of stay is an almost inevitable result.

The case of Mr. S, a 74-year-old man admitted for a transurethral prostatectomy, is an excellent example. Although the physicians and nurses knew that this procedure generally requires a four-day hospital stay and has postoperative restrictions related to driving and lifting, Mr. S was not aware of this information upon admission and for the first three days of his stay. He knew that a friend who had had similar surgery five years earlier had been kept in the hospital for nine days. On the basis of this information, Mr. S suggested to his niece, his major source of support, that she plan her week-long vacation while he was hospitalized because "after all, I'll be in the hospital and you deserve a rest, too." Unfortunately, the clinicians had planned a four-day hospitalization and were then faced with a discharge problem that could have been avoided.

In managed care, clinicians establish the expected length of stay, outcomes, and daily events for the usual patient within a specific case type. This information is then shared with patients and their families either before admission or immediately after admission. The information is further reinforced throughout the health care encounter. For an inpatient admission, reinforcement would occur on a daily basis. Patients and their families then would have an opportunity to incorporate the information into their own plans.

How Managed Care Works

Managed care achieves its benefits by segregating patients according to case type (that is, by presenting diagnosis) and then identifying the patterns that emerge in the care of the case type in terms of outcomes, processes, lengths of stay, resources used, and costs. These patterns of care are identified collaboratively by nurses and physicians. Because the precise sequence of activities is outlined and used during patient care, any deviation from the norm can be identified as it occurs, and problems can be addressed promptly. Early identification and intervention often prevent complications, including prolonged length of stay and increased resource consumption. As a result, managed care also reinforces and strengthens nurses' accountability for moving patients toward outcomes at each shift or encounter.

Initiating Managed Care

As noted earlier, managed care can be implemented in any type of nursing care delivery system, whether it be primary, team, functional, or total patient care. The following four key steps for implementing managed care have been identified as essential to this case management model.

Step 1

The first step is to *specify target case types.* Case types are diagnostic populations (such as myocardial infarction or cholecystectomy patients) that require similar care, use similar amounts and kinds of resources, and have approximately the same length of stay. Although most patients within an institution will eventually be targeted for managed care, it is usually helpful to specify parameters for identifying the initial case types. Such parameters may include the largest case types by volume or cost (or both), case types that are already treated by efficiently functioning multidisciplinary teams, or case types that present problems for the institution for some reason.

Step 2

The next step is to *identify the nurses and physicians who are most familiar with the target case types.* Once the physician-nurse teams have been identified, they outline the time frames within which care will proceed. The time frames include the expected length of stay within all areas in which the patient will receive care (for example, ambulatory, inpatient, operating room), as well as the processes and intermediate goals for each specific time period involved (for example, shift, day, visit, or hour). Because managed care is unit based, the time frames established in this phase allow the caregivers to focus on the parameters for each geographic area.

The usual problems encountered by patients in the target case type are identified by the team. Eventually, standardized terminology will be useful for computerization, but the initial goal should be to develop problem statements on which team members can agree. Problem statements such as those developed by Gettrust and others (1985) may be useful references. A sample problem statement for cerebrovascular accident (CVA) patients would be "Nutrition: potential for less than body requirements."

Step 3

The third step is to *identify expected outcomes of care for each problem.* For example, an expected outcome associated with the problem statement developed in the preceding paragraph might be that the patient "maintain admission weight." Movement toward the outcome is identified by stating intermediate goals by the time period most commonly used in the geographic area (for example, by visit in the ambulatory area or by hour in the emergency room). When possible, intermediate goals are identified for each outcome. Like outcomes, intermediate goals are stated with the patient as the subject. An intermediate goal associated with the outcome stated above may read as follows: "By day 3, the patient takes small sips and/or bites of food and chews thoroughly."

Step 4

The team next *identifies the nursing and physician processes or activities that are necessary to move the patient toward the outcomes and intermediate goals.* A nursing process might be stated as "instructs patient and family regarding signs and symptoms of wound infection and importance of reporting these," while a physician process might state "stabilizes medication regimen and weans patient from unnecessary medications." The processes and intermediate goals are also identified by time periods. Identifying the time periods facilitates a review of the sequence of critical events, such as tests and procedures, to make sure that they are scheduled in an effective, efficient manner.

These four steps provide a clear picture of the current practice patterns used in the care of specific groups of patients. The practice patterns are then reviewed and revised where possible to minimize length of stay and resource utilization while maintaining or improving patient outcomes. The resulting information is formatted into tools known as *case management plans* (the standardized plan of care for patients in a specific diagnostic case type) and *critical paths* (the key incidents that must occur in a predictable and timely fashion to achieve an appropriate length of stay). These tools are more fully described in chapter 4.

Utilizing Managed Care in Daily Practice

As with other patient care delivery systems, managed care uses a defined process (figure 1-2, see p. 19). The managed care process directs the caregiver's attention to outcomes, time frames, and care activities. This process also highlights the shift (or encounter) focus of managed care, another characteristic of this care delivery system.

Daily use of managed care in nursing practice is facilitated by a managed care checklist (figure 1-3, see p. 20). Such a checklist is especially valuable for nursing staff who may be learning about managed care for the first time. It is also supportive to experienced staff members who are making the transition to managed care. The checklist helps them to incorporate managed care concepts into their practice.

Variance Identification

As patients are admitted, the appropriate case management plans and critical paths are selected by the nurse. These are then modified and individualized to meet the needs of the specific patient. This modification is collaboratively accomplished through a review by the nurse and physician. As the patient's care proceeds, actual care is compared with the expected plan of care several times a day in rounds and intershift reports. This results in the identification of variance between expected care and actual care. Variance occurs when the patient's care or progress does not meet the standard or expected care or progress. For example, patients within a specific case type are generally ambulatory by day 2; if a patient is not ambulatory by day 2, this is considered to be a variance.

Three sources of variance have been identified: system, clinician, and patient. System variance occurs when, for example, a Holter monitor is required before the patient is discharged but no monitor is available, resulting in a delayed discharge. An example of clinician variance is found when a hematocrit is required on day 7 but is not ordered or obtained. Patient variance is exemplified by the patient who experiences an intraoperative myocardial infarction, which often results in a prolonged length of stay.

In managed care, nurses are responsible for identifying variance that occurs on their specific shift, for hypothesizing about a cause, and for taking corrective action. As a result of this attention to planned and actual care, variance is identified as it occurs. This is often within sufficient time to effectively reverse negative variance. This system also allows the identification and support of patients who will complete their care in a shorter time frame than projected.

Intershift Report

The process of comparing actual with projected care necessitates changes in nursing systems, primarily in the intershift report. Traditionally, the intershift report focused on the events of the previous 16 hours in the inpatient setting and did not usually direct attention to the status of the patient compared with the expected time frame. In managed care, the report is restructured to compare the patient's actual status with the expected, usual status and to focus the caregiver's attention on the activities that are required during the subsequent shift to move the patient toward anticipated goals.

This approach to the intershift report explicates and strengthens accountability for progress toward outcomes during each shift and enables the care providers, even those who do not consistently provide the patient's care (such as agency, per diem, or part-time nurses), to quickly grasp what needs to be done during their shift or encounter. It also facilitates, especially for intermittent caregivers, a vision of how the work of their shift or encounter contributes to the overall episode of illness. Guidelines for intershift report within a managed care framework are shown in figure 1-4 (see p. 21).

Requisite Nursing Skills/Knowledge

Managed care is most successfully undertaken by nurses who have developed specific supporting skills. A list of these skills is given in figure 1-5 (see p. 22). Although these skills may be acquired through practice in the clinical setting, a theoretical base is also helpful. In addition, nurses new to managed care need basic information about what managed care is and why it is necessary as preparation for fulfilling the case manager's role.

The New England Medical Center Hospitals have developed two specific programs to meet these learning needs. The first is the Staff Nurse Management Program (table 1-1, see p. 23). This program is essential for all new nursing staff, whether or not they are experienced nurses, because it reinforces the concept of nurses as managers and establishes the expectations of the institution. The program outlined in figures 1-6 and 1-7 (see pp. 24–25) is from a curriculum for managed care that takes place over a three- to four-hour time frame. This program, offered to existing nursing staff, provides the curriculum on which phase I of the Staff Nurse Management Program is based.

The delivery of managed care is also predicated on an understanding of the reimbursement structure that is mandated by third-party payers. This suggests that nurses need a working knowledge of prospective payment systems such as diagnosis-related groups (DRGs). Information about reimbursement systems and their effects on health care is available in reference books and programmed instruction texts such as *DRGs: A Programmed Instruction* (Guy and Comeau, 1986). To support the implementation of managed care, nursing departments must implement a system that ensures that each of their staff nurses has access to this information.

☐ Similarities between Case Management and Managed Care

Although case management and managed care involve somewhat different approaches to care, they are mutually supportive and share common goals and characteristics. The goals of these two care modalities (Stetler, 1987) are as follows:

1. To facilitate the achievement of expected or standardized patient outcomes
2. To facilitate early discharge or discharge within an appropriate length of stay
3. To promote appropriate or reduced utilization of resources
4. To promote collaborative practice, coordination of care, and continuity of care
5. To promote professional development and satisfaction of hospital-based registered nurses
6. To direct the contributions of all care providers toward the achievement of patient outcomes

In the process of achieving these goals, managed care and case management also share several characteristics, including a focus on patient outcomes and time frames, an awareness of resource utilization, greater control by patients and clinicians, and a collaborative base. *Outcomes* are defined as aspects of the patient's discharge condition, stated in measurable terms, that result from practitioners' activities. Managed care and case management, then, address the delicate balance between cost, process, outcomes, patient, and practitioner.

□ Differences between Case Management and Managed Care

Although case management and managed care share common goals and characteristics, they approach care somewhat differently. It is useful to explain the differences between case management and managed care by noting that implementing a case management model fundamentally includes all concepts of managed care. The differences between the two are outlined in table 1-2 (see p. 26).

As shown in table 1-2 (see p. 26), the focus shifts from a unit base in managed care to an episode base in case management. In case management, the nurse's accountability extends beyond the geographic unit on which he or she generally practices to the patient's entire episode of illness. In particular, the nurse's accountability is for the outcomes of care that are measured at the completion of the episode of care.

In managed care, the targets of change are the tools and systems of nursing care; that is, the tools and systems are redesigned to facilitate outcome-oriented, cost- and resource-effective care. Case management plans and critical paths are examples of tools that promote managed care; the implementation of group practice typifies a redesigned system. In case management, the target of change is the role of the nurse. The change includes accountability for outcomes throughout the episode of illness as well as responsibility for length of stay and the effective use of resources. Case managers are accountable for working with the physician to develop the expected patterns of care by case type and for reviewing those patterns on a regular basis to ensure that they are accurately reflected in case management plans and critical paths. This process establishes the standards of care for the focus case types. In managed care, some nurses may be asked to develop standards of care by virtue of their expertise in caring for a particular case type. However, the primary responsibility of nurses in managed care is to utilize these tools in their daily care of patients.

Patients within a managed care modality are assigned to nurses at random. For example, primary nurses are usually assigned to patients as their caseload has vacancies. This assignment does not usually focus on a specific patient population. However, in case management, assignment of patients is focused on particular groups of patients, as defined earlier.

In managed care, as in case management, variance is analyzed and outcome achievement is evaluated for individual patients during each shift. However, in case management the case managers also identify, analyze, and take corrective action for the patterns of variance that emerge within their entire caseload over the entire episode of illness. For example, case managers for femoral-popliteal bypass graft patients would identify causes of prolonged length of stay as they occurred over a period of time and among all the patients within that case type. The focus on larger numbers of patients by case types and the identification of patterns of variance facilitate intervention by the case managers within the care system to expedite the patient's care.

Finally, case managers collaborate primarily with specific attending physicians, whereas nurses involved in managed care in teaching hospitals generally collaborate with the house staff.

The case management link with the attending physician is important because the resulting relationship fosters creative approaches to reducing length of stay and resource utilization while focusing on outcomes.

☐ Case Management in the Literature

The literature generally focuses on the implementation of case management in out-of-hospital situations, especially with such target populations as the chronically mentally ill or the elderly or with large groups of individuals, such as those employed by one company. A review of the literature also reveals a number of controversial issues, notably, what the scope of case management is and who case managers should be.

According to the literature, the goals of traditional case management include coordinating services; providing access to resources and services (often discussed under the rubric of "brokerage of services"); controlling costs, especially for high-risk case types (Henderson and Wallack, 1987); and coordinating the health care team (Mazoway, 1987). Many authors include advocacy and quality-related components in their descriptions of case management. However, the literature suggests that the primary focus of case management is to control health care costs.

The question of who should be case managers is one of the most controversial issues in the literature, generating two major questions. The first concerns which health care provider should assume the role. The second concerns the type of relationship that should be established between the patient and the case manager.

As described in the literature, nursing case management is characterized by positioning nurse caregivers as case managers. Although many nurses play a resource-brokering role, the trend is toward exploring roles for nurses as case managers within the context of providing nursing care. In this situation, case management takes place within the care-providing agency. The functions of nursing case management are considered to include assessment, coordination, advocacy, referral, teaching, home visiting, crisis intervention, and medication monitoring (Baier, 1987), most of which are already considered to be within the scope of nursing.

That nurses are uniquely qualified to execute the case manager role is supported by Ethridge (1987, p. 6), who asserts that "the advantage of a nurse is that she not only can coordinate resources but can also deliver direct care and identify those precipitating events that require medical attention. These timely interventions have proven to be not only cost effective but to decrease the fragmentation of multiple providers." Mundinger (1984) agrees, pointing out that nurses can provide the majority of services provided by other types of case managers, but that the reverse is not always true. A combination of nursing and case management skills is especially important in the face of the nursing and medical care needs of case-managed patients.

As in other case management designs, the literature shows that nursing case management has evolved in various directions. The American Nurses' Association (1988) provides a description of several different designs. This diversity of nursing case management models mirrors the diversity within other case management modalities. The consistent thread among all models is the provision of appropriate, cost-effective care to patients.

☐ The Nurse as Case Manager

The model that is described in detail in this book is the nursing caregiver as case manager. Nurses are in a key position to implement case management and managed care by virtue of their clinical skills and the nature of their interactions with patients and other members of the health care team. As Zander (1988, p. 28) observes, "Because of its rich tradition in skilled, compassionate care managed throughout the 24 hours in a day, nursing is in a key position to implement managed care in collaboration with the institution."

In turn, case management promotes a new definition of nursing. This new definition focuses on the outcomes of care as the nursing product while incorporating the tasks and activities that are an integral part of nursing practice. Tasks are viewed within the context of associated outcomes. In nursing case management, case accountability is accomplished by focusing on the desired goals of each shift while having an awareness of the outcomes by case.

As a result of case management, the focus of nursing practice shifts in three dramatic ways:

- From planned to managed care
- From task responsibility to case accountability
- From tasks to outcomes

These shifts are important foundations for a redefinition of nursing care.

☐ *References and Bibliography*

American Nurses' Association. *Case Management: A Challenge for Nurses.* Kansas City, MO: ANA, 1988.

American Nurses' Association. *The Facilitator.* Kansas City, MO: ANA, 1988.

Baier, M. Case management with the chronically mentally ill. *Journal of Psychosocial Nursing* 25(6):17–20, 1987.

Case management is just the ticket for home care. *Hospitals* 60(6), Mar. 20, 1986.

Chollet, D., and Bently, C. Identifying real costs of major illness. *Business and Health* 4(3):14–18, Jan. 1987.

Comeau, E. The nursing product: at what cost? Presented at the National Symposium entitled From Task to Outcome: The Transformation of Professional Nursing. Boston, Apr. 24, 1987.

Daniels, K. Will nurses control care at home? *Home Healthcare Nurse* 6(2): 18–23, 1988.

Deitchman, W. S. How many case managers does it take to screw in a light bulb? *Hospital and Community Psychiatry* 31(11):788–89, 1980.

Downey-DeZell, A., Comeau, E., and Zander, K. Nursing case management: Managed care via the nursing case management model. In: J. Scherubel, editor. *Patients & Pursestrings.* Vol. II. New York City: NLN Publication 20-2191, 1988, pp. 253–64.

Etheredge, M. L., Zander, K., and Bower, K., editors. *Nursing Case Management: Blueprints for Transformation.* Boston: Center for Nursing Case Management, New England Medical Center Hospitals, 1987.

Ethridge, P. Building successful nursing care delivery systems for the future. Paper presented at the National Commission on Nursing Implementation Project Invitational Conference, San Diego, Nov. 4, 1987.

Evashwick, C., Ney, J., and Siemon, J. *Case Management: Issues for Hospitals.* Chicago: American Hospital Association, 1985.

Fisher, K. QA update: case management. *Quality Review Bulletin* 13(8), Aug. 1987.

Franklin, J., Solovitz, B., Mason, M., Clemons, J., and Miller, G. An evaluation of case management. *American Journal of Public Health* 77(6):674–78, 1987.

Freund, D. *Medicaid Reform: Four Studies of Case Management.* Washington, DC: American Enterprise Institute for Public Policy Research, 1984.

Gettrust, K., Ryan, S., and Engleman, D. *Applied Nursing Diagnosis.* New York City: Wiley Medical Publication, 1985.

Goldstrom, I., and Manderscheid, R. A descriptive analysis of community support program case managers serving the chronically mentally ill. *Community Mental Health* 19(1):17–26, 1983.

Grau, L. Case management and the nurse. *Geriatrics,* 1984 [no further publication information available].

Green, G. Case management: state of the art. In: R. Bennet, S. Frisch, B. Gurland, and others, editors. *Coordinated Service Delivery Systems.* New York City: Haworth Press, 1984.

Guy, S., and Comeau, E. *DRGs: A Programmed Instruction.* Boston: Center for Nursing Case Management, New England Medical Center Hospitals, 1986.

Halloran, E., Patterson, C., and Kiley, M. Case-mix: matching patient need with nursing resource. *Nursing Management* 18(3):27–42, 1987.

Hardy, J., King, T., and Repke, J. The Johns Hopkins pregnancy program: an evaluation. *Obstetrics and Gynecology* 69(3), part 1:300–306, 1987.

Harris, M., and Bergman, H. Case management with the chronically mentally ill: a clinical perspective. *American Journal of Orthopsychiatry* 57(2):296–303, 1987.

Health Care Advisory Board. *Nurse Recruitment and Retention.* Washington, DC: Advisory Board Co., 1987.

Henderson, M., Souder, B., and Bergman, A. Measuring efficiencies of managed care. *Business and Health* 4(3):43–46, Jan. 1987.

Henderson, M., and Wallack, S. Evaluating case management for catastrophic illness. *Business and Health* 4(3):7–11, Jan. 1987.

Horowitz, M. Inside the news: case management thrives despite physician protests. *Health Week* 2(6):32–33, 1988.

Iglehart, J. K. Health policy report: Medicaid turns to prepaid managed care. *New England Journal of Medicine* 308(16):976–80, 1983.

Knaus, W., and Wagner, D. When is ICU care appropriate? *Business and Health* 4(3):31–34, Jan. 1987.

Kreiger, G., and Sullivan, J. The case for case management. *Occupational Health and Safety* 56(5):92, 1987.

Lamb, H. R. Therapist-case managers: more than brokers of services. *Hospital and Community Psychiatry* 31(11):762–64, 1980.

Lawler, F., and Hosokawa, M. Evaluation of standards of practice for primary care physicians using 12 hypothetical cases. *Journal of Family Practice* 24(4):377–83, 1987.

Mazoway, J. Early intervention in high-cost care. *Business and Health* 4(3):12–16, Jan. 1987.

McLaughlin, P. Staff nurse management program. In: K. Zander, K. Bower, and M. L. Etheredge. *Handbook of Professional Practice*. Boston: New England Medical Center Hospitals, 1985.

McNiff, M. L. Impact of managed care systems on home health agencies. *Home Healthcare Nurse* 6(2):10-13, 1988.

Merrill, J. Defining case management. *Business and Health* 3(9):5-7, July–Aug. 1985.

Millenson, M. Managed care: will it push providers against the wall? *Hospitals* 60:66, Oct. 5, 1986.

Mundinger, M. O. Community-based care: who will be the case managers? *Nursing Outlook* 32(6):294-95, 1984.

National Commission on Nursing Implementation Project. Second Invitational Conference, San Diego, Nov. 5–6, 1987.

Nursing Assessment and Management of the Frail Elderly (NAMFE). DHHS grant # 5D10NU27069-02. Kansas City, KS: University of Kansas School of Nursing, 1981.

Prottas, J., and Handler, E. The complexities of managed care: operating a voluntary system. *Journal of Health Politics, Policy and Law* 12(2):253-69, 1987.

Roman, M. The critical path. *Success*, Sept. 1987, pp. 56–57 [no further publication information available].

Roper, W. Personal perspective: HCFA sees capitation as the answer to providing affordable health care. *Business and Health* 4(3):64, Jan. 1987.

Rusch, S. Continuity of care: from hospital unit into home. *Nursing Management* 17(12):31-41, 1986.

Schniedman, R., Griffiths, E., and Belock, S. Streamlining care: meeting patient needs through DRGs. *Nursing Success Today* 3(5):23-28, 1986.

Schwartz, S. R., Goldman, H. H., and Churgin, S. Case management for the chronic mentally ill: models and dimensions. *Hospital and Community Psychiatry* 33(12):1006-9, 1982.

Sovie, M. D. Needed now: a hospital partnership for patient care. *Health Care Supervisor* 2(2):27-39, 1984.

St. Amand, L. Managed care: fitting pieces into the puzzle. *Home Healthcare Nurse* 6(2):14-17, 1988.

Stein, J. Costs and care in academic medical centers. *Business and Health* 4(3):50-52, Jan. 1987.

Steinberg, R. M., and Carter, G. W. *Case Management and the Elderly: A Handbook for Planning and Administering Programs*. Lexington, MA: Lexington Books, 1982.

Stetler, C. Preliminary evidence of goal achievement in nursing case management. Presented at the Spring Nursing Forum, New England Medical Center Hospitals, Boston, Mar. 26, 1987. Revised by K. Bower, 1988.

Stetler, C. Case management through collaborative practice: interim report. Unpublished report. Boston: New England Medical Center Hospitals, Department of Nursing, 1988.

Stetler, C., and Downey-Dezell, A. *Case Management Plans: Designs for Transformation.* Boston: Center for Nursing Case Management, New England Medical Center Hospitals, 1987.

Surber, R., Shumway, M., Shadoan, R., and Hargraves, W. Effects of fiscal retrenchment on public mental health services for the chronic mentally ill. *Community Mental Health Journal* 22(3):215–27, 1986.

Wagner, D. Client care management. *Caring* 6(12):12–14, Dec. 1987.

Wahlstedt, P., and Blaser, W. Nurse case management for the frail elderly: a curriculum to prepare nurses for that role. *Home Healthcare Nurse* 4(2):30–35, 1986.

Wright, R., Sklebar, H., and Heiman, J. Patterns of case management activity in an intensive community support program: the first year. *Community Mental Health Journal* 23(1):53–59, 1987.

Zander, K. Managed care within acute care settings: design and implementation via nursing case management. *Health Care Supervisor* 6(2):27–43, 1988.

Zander, K. Nursing case management: resolving the DRG paradox. *Nursing Clinics of North America* 23(3), Sept. 1988.

Zander, K. Nursing case management: strategic management of cost and quality outcomes. *Journal of Nursing Administration* 18(5):23–30, 1988.

Figure 1-1. Connecting Outcomes, Cost, and Process

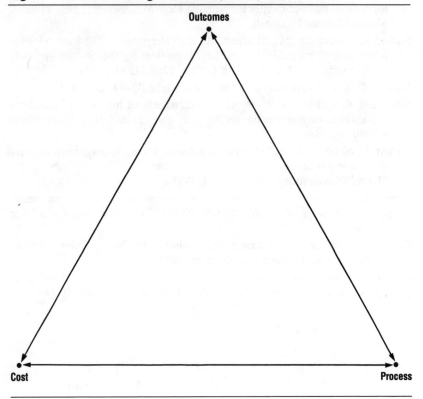

Figure 1-2. The Managed Care Process

1. Assess the patient, focusing on the current needs for care and exploring after care needs and resources.

2. Select, review, and adapt the case management plan and critical path to the individual patient.
   - Note the DRG and discharge/transfer dates.
   - Insert the critical path in the nursing kardex.
   - Highlight the expected outcomes.

3. Structure the work of the shift and intershift report to focus on the expected critical events.

4. Note negative variances encountered in the critical path. Seek consultation.

5. Evaluate and document progress toward expected outcomes and variances encountered.
   - Note variances on the back of the critical path.
   - Hypothesize about why the variance occurred, focusing on issues germane to the system, the practitioners, or the patient.

6. Introduce self as the caregiver and review plans for the shift with the patient.

7. At discharge, review the case, focusing on the outcomes (Were they realistic and met?), processes (Did they lead to outcomes efficiently and effectively?) and variances encountered.

Source: Copyright, New England Medical Center Hospitals, 1987. Developed by K. Bower.

Figure 1-3. Managed Care Checklist

1. Is there a critical path in the nursing kardex? _____

2. Do I know the anticipated discharge date for each of the patients I am caring for this shift? _____

3. Do I know what the expected, standardized outcomes are for each of the patients I am caring for? _____

4. Do I know the critical events that should occur today to move my patients toward the expected outcomes within the anticipated length of stay? _____

5. Do I introduce myself to my assigned patients and review plans for the day? _____

6. In report do I provide and receive information about:

   • Anticipated length of stay and day of length of stay (for example, day 6 of an estimated 9-day stay) _____

   • Critical events anticipated for today and the next shift _____

   • Difficulties in moving toward outcomes _____

   • Variances from the expected timeline _____

   • Anticipated DRG _____

7. Do I seek consultation and note when negative variances occur? _____

8. Do I provide documentation about the anticipated length of stay, outcomes, and progress toward them? _____

Source: Copyright, New England Medical Center Hospitals, 1987. Developed by K. Bower.

Figure 1-4. Managed Care Guidelines for Intershift Report

Patient name

Diagnosis, anticipated length of stay, and DRG number

Brief medical and social history

Patient day number (for example, day 2 of a 5-day stay)

Patient's present condition and critical activities identified on the critical path expected for that day (for example, visit from the ostomy nurse, ambulate three times a day, and so forth).

Evaluation of compliance with the critical path and potential or actual reasons for lack of compliance with the critical path (for example, pain management issues such as prolonged use of intramuscular narcotics). If reasons are unclear, a case consultation should be scheduled.

Source: Copyright, New England Medical Center Hospitals, 1987. Developed by J. G. Somerville.

Figure 1-5. Managed Care Skills Checklist

Assessment, case specific
   Initial
   Ongoing

Use of critical paths

Outcome identification

Variance identification

Variance analysis

Identification of goals for shift

Focus care towards shift goals and outcomes

Prediction of patient needs beyond the immediate shift

Follow-up documentation of:
   Progress towards outcomes
   Variance identified

Identification of issues for case consultation

Collaboration with:
   Physicians
   Other health care team members

Identification of patients' discharge needs

Resources (including payer benefits)

Negotiation

Communication: Use of report for managed care

Running a health care team meeting

Source: Copyright, New England Medical Center Hospitals, 1987.

Table 1-1. Staff Nurse Management Program

This program has been designed to assist the staff nurse in the New England Medical Center System to understand his or her role as primary nurse in managed care, shift charge nurse, and case manager. The program is divided into three phases, with each phase concentrating on role-related topics. It is also designed with practice sessions to assist nurses in assessing their abilities in managerial situations.

Phase I	Phase II	Phase III
• All staff RNs entering NEMC.	• Staff RNs working on general units.	• Staff RNs working on general units.
• 6–8 weeks.	• Staff RNs at the 3–6-month level.	• Staff RNs at the 6–12-month level.
• All-day class.	• All-day seminar.	• All-day seminar.
• Overview of managed care. Each phase of the nursing process is paralleled with concepts of managed care.	• Seminar spotlights roles of shift charge nurse and case manager. Seminar reviews the tasks, management skills required, and the NEMC resources available to staff nurse.	• Seminar provides the opportunity to analyze and practice management theories and skills through individual as well as group exercises.
• Skills: complete DRG posttest.	• Skills: communication, priority setting, decision making, planning, problem solving, delegation, and organization.	• Skills: cooperation, conflict, confrontation, negotiation, power, and influence.
• Common issues discussed: a. Discharge planning b. Legislation c. Resources d. Home assessments e. Case consultation	• Common issues related to charge nurse role: a. Making assignments based on staff's job description b. Utilizing resources c. Lack of confidence with delegation and follow-up d. Being part of the problem-solving system	• Common issues discussed: a. How to approach staff (MD, peer, ancillary) when a conflict occurs b. Uncertainty of how to use the problem-solving process for broader unit issues c. Feeling powerless to change existing problem situations

Source: Reprinted, with permission, from McLaughlin, P. In Zander, K., Bower, K., and Etheredge, M. L. *Handbook of Professional Practice.* Boston: New England Medical Center Hospitals, 1985, p. 210.

Figure 1-6. Managed Care Program Objectives

Purpose:

The purpose of this program is to define managed care within the context of the primary nursing role; to introduce participants to the tools and practices for managing care; and to initiate the ongoing use of the tools for managed care for patient care and shift report.

Objectives:

At the completion of this program, the participant will be able to:

1. Define managed care as a way of reorganizing systems to maximize control that the nurse at the bedside has in delivering care.

2. Identify the elements of the managed care process.

3. Cite environmental forces mandating a transition to managed care.

4. Describe the tools available to manage care and describe how these tools are utilized in daily practice.

5. Demonstrate how systems have been redesigned to support managed care.

6. Identify the skills required for managed care.

Source: Developed by K. Bower and M. L. Etheredge, New England Medical Center Hospitals, 1988.

Figure 1-7. Managed Care Sample Program Schedule for Staff

Managed Care: An Outcome Driven Model
- Why Managed Care: Environmental Forces
- Managed Care Defined
- Elements of the Managed Care Process
- Benefits of Managed Care
- Tapping into the Pareto Principle

Retooling the Production Process
- Case Management Plans: Defining Our Business
- Critical Paths
- Identifying and Analyzing Variance

Redesigning Systems: Making Them Work for Patients and Nurses
- Shift Report
- Rounds
- Health Care Team Meeting
- Case Consultation

Skills for Managed Care
- Extending the Horizon: Moving toward Case Management

Source: Developed by New England Medical Center Department of Nursing, 1988.

Table 1-2. Comparison of Managed Care and Case Management

Characteristic	Managed Care	Case Management
Focus	Unit	Episode
Changes	Tools and systems	Nurse's role
Patient assigned by	Random	Case type/attending physician
Evaluation	Individual patients	Aggregate patients
MD collaboration	House staff/attending physician	Attending physician
Variance identified	Shift Individual patient	Shift and episode Individual patient and aggregate patients

Source: Copyright, New England Medical Center Hospitals, 1988.

Designing the Nurse Case Manager's Role

Because case management changes the role of the staff nurse, it is important to understand how the role is designed and how it affects both unit functioning and the individual staff nurse. This chapter describes various configurations of the nurse case manager's role as well as its impact on the hospital environment.

☐ Creating a Patient-Centered Matrix

In nursing case management, the accountability for clinical and cost outcomes per patient rests with the nurse case manager. This accountability is achieved through continuity of plan between nurses throughout the entire episode of care, coordination of resources, and collaboration with the attending physician. To accomplish such a broad undertaking, the primary nurse/staff nurse case manager is placed in a matrix at the direct patient care level.

In this case-based matrix, the staff nurse works individually with the physician(s) and, as a member of a multiunit nursing group, with the physician(s) in a formal group practice. The nurse case manager is a member of a unit-based staff and a member of the group practice.

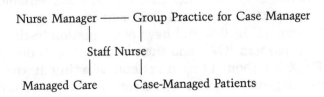

```
Nurse Manager ——— Group Practice for Case Manager
       |             |
            Staff Nurse
       |             |
Managed Care   Case-Managed Patients
```

As in other matrix organizations, a "matrix demands new behavior, attitudes, skills, and knowledge" because people are expected to function in new ways (Davis and Lawrence, 1977, p. 103). In essence, a matrix creates new interdependencies that necessitate new communication patterns within the institution. Of course, in health care the interdependencies have always existed but rarely have been given formal structures. Case management imposes a structure and commitment on the strategic management of cost and quality outcomes. Understanding case management as a formal patient-centered matrix within the institutional setting is helpful in implementing this model.

Group Practice Configuration

Group practice is an integral part of the case management model because all case-managed patients are assigned upon admission to a formally prepared group practice. There are many possible ways to configure a group practice. For instance, the common denominator may be the attending physician, a group of attending physicians, a case type, a referring agency, an insurance plan, or a category of patient (such as geriatric). From these possible configurations, two predominant patterns emerge: cluster and serial.

Cluster Configuration

The cluster is more frequently used when one physician or agency admits a patient to one unit and then that patient is discharged to the referring physician or agency. The group practice determines who among the principals is in the best situation to assume the case manager role for each patient who enters the group practice. This decision is made at the time of the patient's admission to the group practice and is determined by past commitments and contacts with the patient, anticipated hospital course, scheduling, and other case type-specific variables.

For example, all patients of Dr. X admitted for transurethral prostatectomy (TURP) would have preadmission testing, go to the operating room (OR), and then be assigned to one of four units. Dr. X has about 12 such patients at a time in the hospital, and so the group practice would consist of an operating room or recovery room nurse (if possible) and one nurse from each of the four units. The assigned nurse would give care to Dr. X's TURP patients using Dr. X's TURP critical path, within his or her shift and caseload. Each nurse would be educated specifically about TURP and would meet weekly with other nurses in the group practice and with Dr. X on a regular basis. The configuration can be illustrated as follows:

Dr. X —→ Preadmission —→ OR
Unit A (3 patients)
Unit B (3 patients)
Unit C (3 patients)
Unit D (3 patients)
—→ Home

Another example of the cluster configuration could be shown by having all nonsurgical patients from Green Manor Nursing Home, regardless of case type or physician, admitted to one of two acute care units. There are usually five of these patients at any time. One nurse from Unit A and one from Unit B, using critical paths and working with the physician coverage, take Green Manor Nursing Home patients in their shift and caseload, as illustrated below:

Nursing home
Unit A (4 patients)
Unit B (1 patient)
→ Nursing home

Serial Configuration

The serial configuration applies to patients who will predictably go through several units, such as patients with multiple trauma. In large hospitals, up to 40 of these patients at a time may be somewhere in the system, often distributed among the air or ground transport unit, the emergency department (ED), the operating room, and in some instances, the intensive care unit (ICU); an orthopedic, neurology, or postoperative surgical unit; and a rehabilitation unit:

Air/ground transport —→ ED —→ OR
Ortho unit
Neuro unit
Surgical unit
—→ Rehabilitation/Home

In the serial configuration, one physician usually specializes in a particular case type. Except for the transport nurse, the nurses have not specialized and have not met many of the other nurses throughout the institution who share their patients. Case management and group practice give them a chance to gain specialty training within their generalist positions without having to change jobs. This particular group practice might begin with three nurses from each area represented. It could eventually develop sophisticated education and communication networks among the nurses, among the nurses and physicians, and especially among all the members and the patients and families.

In the future, the serial configuration may extend into other agencies within the larger health care system. For instance, a stroke patient ready to leave the acute care unit might move to an extended care facility (ECF) before beginning active rehabilitation. Such a patient might be cared for by a member of a nursing group practice even though the physician might change. For example:

Acute care ⟶ ECF ⟶ Rehabilitation ⟶ Home

This kind of coordination facilitates movement into and out of appropriate units. In addition, for the patient and family, it provides the security of knowing that the standards of care of one department will be maintained by the next.

☐ Selection of Case Types

Case management can usually be implemented effectively with a defined group of patients managed by a specific set of physicians and nurses working in a group practice. In other words, it is "business as usual" for most patients, with case management applied only to a limited number of patients. Nursing continues its care delivery systems around the clock, and physicians continue their clinical practices. Case management reframes, refocuses, and realigns these two groups without directly affecting work-load assignments.

In selecting the case types with which to begin case management, it is advantageous to determine the extent of involvement that an institution currently has or desires to have with those types of patients. Generally, case types that are catastrophic in nature (such as leukemia patients or neonates) are selected to receive case management first because there is usually a clear beginning for treatment (for example, a patient with myocardial infarction coming to the ED) and a clear end (discharge, transfer, or death). For best results, however, this decision, as well as all others about case management, should be made with the active input of clinicians, especially those who understand the case management model, rather than solely by hospital administrators.

The next step is for the physicians, nurses, and staff from other departments instrumental to the smooth flow of care for patients in the selected case types to develop case management plans and critical paths. The institution should supply all financial, length-of-stay, and quality assurance data available. As appropriate patterns of care are outlined on these protocols, the role of each participant is clarified. Using this technique, the clinicians and administrators become patient centered rather than department centered, and roles are designed as a means to an end rather than as an end in themselves. Through this method, flexibility, creativity, and collaboration are stimulated.

☐ The Role of the Case Manager: Key to Successful Implementation

The staff nurse case manager is the person who makes the system work for patients, families, and physicians. Because the case manager is also a primary caregiver, he or she is in a key position to adapt policies and procedures and to note any variance in the patient's progress as determined by the critical path.

Definition of Role

The nurse case manager is a professional nurse who is responsible for a comprehensive assessment of the patient's current condition; the setting of potential outcomes and plans to meet these outcomes in collaboration with the patient, family, and physician; and the ongoing coordination, monitoring, and evaluation of actions taken on the patient's behalf. The role begins when the patient enters the system and ends when accountability is transferred to specific people or agencies beyond the legal and financial bounds of the institution.

For example, for some case types, the case manager's role begins and ends within one building, one or two units, and one admission. For other case types, the involvement may be long and intense. Case management may last for four days, as with a patient undergoing prostatectomy, or for four years, as with a patient who has diabetes.

Description of Role

The role of the nurse case manager includes the following responsibilities:

- To establish a mechanism for notification when a new patient enters the caseload (this includes determining which patients he or she will manage)
- To introduce self to the patient, the patient's family, or both, and to explain the role of the case manager and group practice
- To give the patient and family the group practice business card
- To contact the physician(s) to begin sharing assessments, goals, and plans for this patient's episode of illness
- To know the anticipated diagnosis-related group (DRG), length of stay, and transfer/discharge dates
- To discuss ongoing and future care with the other nursing staff on the units (inpatient and ambulatory) to which the patient will most likely be transferred
- To negotiate work schedule with the nurse manager (head nurse) to attend weekly group practice meetings
- To compare the standard case management plan with the patient's individual needs in such areas as social and economic data, family resources, functional abilities, knowledge needs, potential risk factors and complications, and special issues
- To identify a critical path for the patient and place it in the nursing kardex
- To review and revise the individual critical path with the physician within 24 hours of admission

- To contact other key members of each patient's team (for example, the social worker, dietitian, physical therapist, community resources personnel, and others, as needed)
- To give and monitor the delivery of care and the patient's responses to care every day that the patient is on the case manager's unit
- To arrange for continuity of plan and provide coverage during short, long, and unexpected absences
- To give the patient and family a time schedule and tell them whom to contact in the case manager's absence
- To document the achievement of intermediate goals and clinical outcomes as they occur
- To integrate case management information and revised interventions (processes) into intershift report and group practice meetings
- To request consultation and feedback before a crisis occurs
- To plan, participate in, and follow through with health care team meetings as needed
- To manage each patient's transitions through the system and transfer accountability to the appropriate person or agency upon discharge
- To complete a follow-up evaluation

As much as possible, potential case managers should be helped to understand the responsibilities of the role as well as the parameters of the commitment. The following questions are useful in defining the boundaries of the case manager's role:

- Is this an experimental or permanent role change?
- Is this a promotion or an extension of current responsibilities?
- Is flexible time or compensatory time involved? How are other responsibilities covered or redistributed? How will the case manager be evaluated?
- What is the off-unit time involved?
- What conference, home visit, and other out-of-hospital responsibilities are involved?
- What computer, secretarial, and other supports are available?

The answers to these questions may not always come readily. The role change for a nurse who functions as a case manager must be evaluated in conjunction with the other aspects of the nurse's role and with those of nonnursing personnel in the health care setting.

Criteria for Selection

Once the baseline roles and the clinical areas involved in each case type have been determined, the staff nurses who will serve as case managers are selected. The selection process is primarily the responsibility of the nurse manager (head nurse) who oversees the day-to-day activities of the case managers in his or her unit. Ideally, all staff nurses who act as case managers should have a master's degree in nursing, take an updated course in physical assessment, and have many years of experience in a specialized field. However, this is neither practical nor necessary when a good curriculum and ongoing support services are in place for the new case managers and the group practices.

Educational preparation is a complicated issue because case management is not formally taught in basic nursing programs at this time. The American Nurses' Association recommends that the minimal preparation for a nurse case manager be a baccalaureate degree in nursing with one year's clinical experience. Fuszard and others (1988, p. 8) suggest the following educational approach:

> The graduate of a baccalaureate program in nursing is prepared to synthesize relevant information, make clinical inferences, project patient outcomes, establish care plans to reach those outcomes, and evaluate the patient's response to nursing interventions. This educational approach prepares the nurse to learn how to function as case manager in group practice with other health care professionals in both institutional and community settings.

The initial implementation at New England Medical Center has shown that clinical experience and an above-average evaluation as a primary nurse are the most valuable qualifications for a case manager. Although most of the staff nurses involved in case management do have a bachelor's degree in nursing, a proven track record as an effective primary nurse can serve as an equivalent qualification. This equivalency must include: (a) knowledge and use of the nursing process, (b) collaborative relationships with physicians and patients/families, and (c) excellent management skills as demonstrated by management of self, shifts (as charge nurse), and caseloads.

Recruiting nurse case managers from within the institution is preferable because a recruiter reviewing outside candidates would need to rely heavily on references to screen candidates for case management positions. In addition to the academic and practice criteria already stated, the recruiter would need to assess the candidate for a track record of (a) taking initiative and following through with complex problems, (b) having effective communication skills, (c) possessing the ability to be either a follower or a leader in groups, and (d) showing interest in the welfare of the institution and the community it serves.

Anyone embarking on case management should be able to work interdependently in situations that are sometimes highly ambiguous. Potential case managers should be interested in the case management model and be ready to make a new level of commitment to patients, colleagues, and the well-being of the institution. "Greater emotional energy is required because people must be open, take more risks, work at developing trust and trusting others" (Davis and Lawrence, 1977, p. 108).

☐ New Role Relationships: Implications for Change

Case management, in general, is a major set of role renegotiations, which begin with the staff nurse's role. The establishment of a case management model raises questions about the case manager's role in relation to other staff and departments, as well as questions about the impact on the overall functioning of the institution. For instance:

- *What is the relationship of the case manager to house staff and attending physicians?* Because the case manager as a staff nurse deals with the day-to-day details of patient care, the case manager must maintain good working relationships with all house staff. The case manager will probably have had an ongoing collegial relationship with the attending physicians and will at times need to describe or clarify the rationale for certain requests made of the house staff. The house staff will regard the case manager as an experienced clinician and provide support.

- *What is the case manager's authority in relation to professionals from social services, dietary, pharmacy, and other departments?* The case manager has as much authority with other departments as he or she is willing to assert in the patient's best interest. When other departments that are key to the smooth management of care are involved in the design of critical paths and the evaluation of variances, each department in effect grants authority to the process of case management.

- *What is the case manager's authority in relation to nursing colleagues on his or her unit, as well as to nurses in the group practice from other units?* Because the case manager is accountable for clinical outcomes and lengths of stay, he or she is (theoretically) the authority on the nursing care of specific patients within the group practice. However, this authority must be constantly earned with one's nursing colleagues, regardless of title. The confidence that results from being a member of a group practice helps each staff nurse to use authority in appropriate, effective ways.

- *How does case management affect product line management (that is, patient care and outcomes), quality assurance, continuing care departments, program planning, and so forth?* Case management positively affects other systems and programs in acute care because it is done with an accurate understanding of the production process on the part of everyone involved. Continuing care is used on a more timely basis, and quality assurance is implemented concurrently by the clinicians actually providing the care. Both program planning and product line management will be strengthened as a result of the clinical and financial predictability introduced by clinical paths and the linchpin function of group practices.

- *How can case management improve admitting and discharge practices, patient education and support programs, marketing, and so forth!* For the reasons already stated, case management improves a hospital's caregiving process. Because of the model's design and the collaboration it engenders, actual clinical practice is improved, as is the institution's ability to receive accurate feedback about the effectiveness of its systems, such as admitting and education. Of course, to achieve solid change, the entire administration must be willing to respond to these data long past the initial stresses of implementation. Once the institution feels confident in its ability to produce identifiable cost and quality outcomes, the best marketing tools will be the clinicians and patients themselves.

What is the worth of case management to the institution! The worth of any change as profound as prospective reimbursement and case management is still unclear; preliminary data are positive but not conclusive. However, there is enormous worth in any process that finally identifies physicians and nurses as accountable for the financial and clinical outcomes of patients and institutionally assists them in this endeavor by providing better tools, systems, and relationships with which to do their work. Anyone in health care knows how much effort it takes for a case to go smoothly. Case management unites the four main parties — administrators, physicians, nurses, and patients and their families — in an approach that has its foundation in common sense. Onlookers wonder why we have not done this sooner.

The role of group practice in case management may also draw questions from those not familiar with the concept. For example:

- *Is group practice as defined in case management the same as team nursing!* No. Team spirit and team building are part of group practice, but members of group practice are just as well prepared as registered staff nurses who share the same set of patients. They each give the patient care when the patient is in their unit. Each nurse provides direct care for the same number of patients he or she had before case management was instituted. The nurse who is case manager for a specific patient is given that responsibility by his or her own group. That nurse works collaboratively with peers on the unit and colleagues in the group.

- *What incentives do physicians have to become involved?* The nursing group practice drafts the details of the case management plans and critical paths, which are then reviewed and validated by key physicians. Physicians are concerned with the safety and the satisfaction of their patients, and they want timely information about their progress. With the consistency of nursing care that group practice and the use of critical paths provide, physicians develop more confidence in the way patients are managed. They may not come to all meetings, but they can be more involved in ways developed among themselves and the nurses.

- *Isn't this adding a layer to the bureaucracy?* No extra administrative layer is required. The group practice is composed of nurse and physician caregivers who are managing their cases. All they require is time to coordinate their activities and better management tools, documentation, and information systems.

As in every role redesign effort, the initial theory and "buy-in" are just the beginning of a complex process. Roles in patient care are, in truth, renegotiated and "redesigned" with every contact between care providers and their patients. The change toward a focus on outcomes within a time frame gives direction to the care providers, but also begins a chain of events throughout the institution that needs to be consistently monitored by managers and administrators.

☐ *References*

Davis, S., and Lawrence, P. *Matrix.* Reading, MA: Addison-Wesley Publishing Co., 1977.

Fuszard, B., and others. *Case Management—A Challenge for Nurses.* Kansas City, MO: American Nurses' Association, 1988.

Educational Preparation for Nurse Case Managers and Nurse Managers/Supervisors

Case management is an advanced set of skills and processes for nursing. As such, the nurses who become case managers need skill development and information to become effective in the role. Similarly, the individuals who manage the case managers must also develop new skills and acquire new information.

An effective curriculum improves the working relationships and practice patterns between physicians and nurses, which in turn can dramatically affect cost and quality outcomes. Although it would be ideal to include physicians in all classroom activities, establishing case management does not depend on that. Instead, providing a curriculum to staff nurses who will become case managers and using case management plans and critical paths collaboratively designed with physicians is a reasonable place to begin.

☐ Case Management Curriculum for Nurse Case Managers

The educational development of staff nurse case managers is vital to a smooth role transition. Although curricula must be custom designed to some degree for each institution, many fundamental areas are common to all settings. The courses cover helping clinicians to integrate management skills with their everyday work.

Certain basic content is included in all case management curricula:

1. The rationale for case management: an overview of changes in the industry
2. The nursing process (advanced level)
3. Case type–specific knowledge
4. System-specific knowledge
5. Collaboration and team building

Both the curriculum and the teaching methods should be designed to stimulate cognitive, affective, and psychomotor development (Gronlund, 1978). Cognitive development is stimulated by building connections between various kinds of information. Affective development, or values and feelings, is promoted by active student involvement in and out of class. Psychomotor development requires the application of cognitive and technical skills to a task or problem.

The best curricula unite all three areas toward an objective, although not necessarily simultaneously. For example, if one objective is to have each nurse assume responsibility for resource allocation, then the curriculum must include (1) the definition of resource allocation with specific examples from the nurse's practice (cognitive domain), (2) the rationale for and feelings about this new role responsibility (affective domain), and (3) a review of an actual case or case study to determine the consequences of actions taken in relation to resource allocation (psychomotor domain). Sample objectives in each domain for participants in a case management curriculum are given in the appendix at the end of this book.

Case management is easier to teach, of course, when the institution, as reflected by the attitudes of the staff nurses, is predisposed to change. Unfortunately, this attitude is not always prevalent in health care agencies even though roles, traditions, and mind-sets have never been as widely challenged as they are today. A useful text, especially for the people developing a case management curriculum, is *Thriving on Chaos* by Tom Peters (1987). One of Peters's many salient points is that, for many industries today, training and retraining staff is a necessity.

☐ Requisite Background Knowledge

Three practice elements should be considered prerequisites to the three-day curriculum described in this chapter. They are (1) a staff nurse management program, (2) a philosophy of comfort in commitment, and (3) DRG literacy.

Staff Nurse Management Program

The staff nurse management program is designed to introduce the staff nurse to the basic skills necessary to manage a caseload of primary patients and to function as a shift charge nurse. The staff nurse management program can easily be expanded to include managed care concepts and an overview of the case manager's role, including a review of the tools utilized by the case manager. As described in chapter 1, the program is divided into three phases—primary nurse in managed care, shift charge nurse, and management skill development—with each phase concentrating on role-related topics. Attendance at each session is mandatory for each new nurse entering the system. The staff nurse management program should be completed within the first year of employment.

Comfort in Commitment

Staff nurses who work in institutions that have a primary nursing model firmly in place should have experience in carrying an average caseload of three to four primary patients at any one time. In the case management program, patients are assigned to a primary nurse on or before admission to a unit, and every nurse is a primary nurse at all times. The nurse, patient, and family all understand the commitment and regularly discuss their expectations of each other.

Primary nurses know that they are accountable for the clinical outcomes achievable by the end of the patient's stay on their units. Nursing documentation and weekly case consultation reinforce this role. Primary nurses learn how to stay professionally close to patients without tipping the balance toward overinvolvement or underinvolvement (Peplau, 1980). Professionally close commitments to patients as well as to the nursing unit and department support for primary nursing build accountability into the fabric of every primary nurse's role.

Institutions that have not fully developed primary nursing as their professional model must devote a concerted effort to the establishment of accountability. The inculcation of accountability is a long-term process that can be accelerated by case management but must be supported concretely by several factors within an institution. These factors include the following: (1) developing a consensus about the specific clinical outcomes for which the primary nurse is accountable, (2) determining a manageable caseload to which the nurse is assigned as part of his or her shift assignment, (3) monitoring the degree of professional closeness and responding to nurses' needs for consultation, and (4) continuously encouraging nurses to take initiative, to risk collaboration, and to fairly evaluate each other's interventions.

DRG Literacy

The financial constraints of the prospective payment system made on the basis of diagnosis-related groups (DRGs) have forced hospitals to look for ways to cut costs. In some instances, nursing departments have suffered. However, it is clear that prospective payment systems are here to stay and that they will have a major impact on the U.S. health care system.

Because nurses and physicians allocate as much as 80 percent of a hospital's resources, the staff nurse can have a significant impact on the cost of care. The staff nurse has more contact with the patient than any other member of the health care team and has 24-hour, seven-day-a-week accountability for achieving patient outcomes. She or he is also in the best position to coordinate the way the other departments in the hospital affect patient care. Thus, the primary nurse/staff nurse is also able to have a significant impact on length of stay.

It is essential that staff nurses understand DRGs and their implications, both negative and positive, for nursing. As a case manager, the primary nurse identifies the expected patient outcomes and is in charge of the nursing process required to produce those outcomes. Each case manager should know the probable DRG for her or his primary patients and the length of stay and resource utilization for that DRG. The case management plan incorporates that information, and the nursing process determined to produce the outcomes includes a time frame for each step of the process.

DRG-programmed instruction, based on behavioral objectives, clarifies the level of knowledge to be attained (Gronlund, 1978). For example, each primary nurse in the New England Medical Center Hospitals (NEMCH) system is expected to demonstrate DRG literacy by meeting the following objectives (Guy and Comeau, 1986):

Level: Introduction
Clarifier: Knowledge
• States a brief history of DRGs nationally and in Massachusetts
• Explains why DRGs and their possible sequels are here to stay
• Defines diagnosis-related group (DRG), length of stay (LOS), and major diagnostic category
• Describes NEMCH's response to DRGs

Level: Familiarization
Clarifier: Comprehension
• Explains what DRGs have to do with specific primary patients in a nurse's caseload in relation to DRGs, LOS, and costs

Level: Competency
Clarifier: Application
• States how a nurse's primary patients are assigned and charged per DRG
• Describes different DRG management reports available for case managers in clinical areas

The programmed instruction can be used in several ways: to orient new clinicians, to provide continuing education for experienced health care managers and clinicians, and to instruct students in clinical and administrative undergraduate and graduate programs. A posttest is provided, and continuing education units (CEUs) are awarded upon successful completion.

□ Case Management Educational Series

The case management curriculum described in the following paragraphs (developed by Zander and Stetler, 1987) is offered as a three-day educational series over a three-week period. It can, of course, be augmented and extended (particularly to include the prerequisite practice elements previously described), but it probably cannot be condensed. The curriculum is offered to specific nurses chosen by their nurse managers to be members of group practices. It is helpful to send each participant an introductory letter and a packet of materials before the first class. This packet should include:

- Class schedule
- Reading list
- Ground rules for case management
- All issues of *Definition* (a quarterly newsletter published by the Center for Nursing Case Management)
- Case study titled "The No-Care Zone" (Loth, 1987)

Adjusting staffing schedules to ensure attendance during work time and awarding CEUs upon completion of each day's program indicate that nurse managers and the institution as a whole are committed to the program and give it the highest priority.

The following outline is an overview of the topics covered in the case management educational series (developed by K. Zander and C. Stetler):

Day One
  (Administer Pretests)
    I. Introducing case management
      A. Definition and rationale
      B. Case management background
      C. NEMCH model
    II. Defining our business
      A. Case management plans
      B. Critical paths
      C. Moving from planned care to managed care
   III. Defining the group practice
      A. Identifying the RNs, MDs, and patients
      B. Team building (Focus: to identify the group practice members)

IV. Updating assessment skills
  A. Physical assessment—new importance
  B. Functional assessment—new base
  C. Family assessment—new team
  D. Case type–specific issues
V. Team-building assignment

Day Two
  (Review Assignment)
  I. Realistic outcomes within time frames
    A. Predicting and individualizing outcomes from experience
    B. Reimbursement and continuing care
    C. Helping your patient survive at home
  II. Case type–specific variances
    A. Complications due to extension of the disease process
    B. Complications related to treatment
    C. Complications unrelated to treatment
  III. Team building (Focus: to identify the work of the group practice)
  IV. RN–MD collaboration
    A. Five building blocks of collaborative practice
    B. How to run a health care team meeting
  V. Assignment

Day Three
  (Review Assignment)
  I. Concurrent review
    A. Tracking and documenting care
    B. Use of telephone
    C. How to provide case consultation to peers
  II. Formal evaluation
    A. Identifying trends for groups of patients
    B. Using research and resources
    C. Changing systems
  III. Landmarks of a well-functioning group
    A. Case example
    B. Team building (Focus: to identify how the group practice continues to develop)

☐ Preparation of Head Nurses and Supervisors

Because nurse managers (head nurses) facilitate case management at the operational level, without their support and creativity case management would be difficult if not impossible to accomplish. The role of the nurse manager is multifaceted in its support of the practice of case management on the unit level. To be successful, the focus of the entire nursing staff must change:

- From an eight-hour shift to an episode of illness
- From planning care to managing care
- From performing tasks to meeting patient outcomes

Introducing the concept to members of the multidisciplinary team, interpreting the purpose of the model, and providing direction to team members are critical functions of the nurse manager. The purpose of case management must be consistently and continually reinforced. This purpose, of course, is not to dictate care, but to outline patterns of care. The idea that tools do not represent standing orders requires constant reinforcement.

Once the nurse manager has interviewed and appointed the staff nurses who will serve as case managers, the role of the nurse manager shifts to developing and supporting the role of case manager by performing the following functions:

- *Adjusting time schedules* to accommodate the case manager's attendance at group practice meetings (this may mean the nurse manager personally covers the case manager's on-unit assignment so that this goal can be accomplished)
- *Providing appropriate resource and educational opportunities* to develop the case manager's knowledge base (this

includes on-unit staff development, participation in the case management curriculum, accessibility of case management plans, critical paths, DRG information, and so forth)
- *Providing consultation* to the case manager and/or acting as a facilitator of a group practice

The themes for management education center on setting a daily structure, developing and coaching staff, and evaluating clinical outcomes. Examples of specific learning needs center on answers to the following questions:

1. How should supervisors manage staff members whose boundaries are beginning to extend beyond the unit base? This situation presents unique challenges and requires new approaches to managing time.
2. What systems are needed to support case management and case managers, and how can they be developed? For example, what system will enable case managers to have pre-hospitalization information and contact with their patients?
3. How should case managers be selected, prepared, and developed?
4. How should case management be evaluated and audited on the unit?
5. How do case managers analyze variances for individual patients?
6. How should group practices be facilitated?

□ Developing the Nursing Case Management Model

This section presents syllabus content that focuses on developing the nursing case management model. The model was developed at NEMCH over a two-year period in a series of monthly seminars attended by all of the nursing department's management staff. The first phase of model development was begun in 1985 and consisted of case type analysis projects designed to focus the nurse manager's attention on resource utilization, length of stay, and practice patterns for a specific case type. The next phase, begun in 1986, focuses on implementing case management.

Management Training Seminars

The following sections describe goals and background for management training seminars and tell how to conduct a case type analysis project and subsequently implement a case management system.

Background

Every member of the nursing department's management staff is required to attend a 90-minute seminar each month. The topics presented at NEMCH seminars in 1986 are shown in table 3-1 (see p. 54) and those presented in 1987 are shown in figure 3-1 (see pp. 55–56). Several seminars are held during the month so that every management staff member is able to attend a seminar in a group with his or her peers. For example, all the evening supervisory staff attend a seminar together. The nurse managers (head nurses) are divided into three groups. The chairman and vice-chairman of nursing attend all seminars.

The teaching methodology for the seminars varies. Didactic teaching and small-group problem-solving sessions are useful methodologies. However, the consultation process is most frequently used. Educating the management staff about the consultation process enables them to present a problem or issue for consultation. Experiential learning on how to be consultants to one's peers is a valuable strategy. The consultant and the consultee follow specific protocols for presentation. In addition to seminar time, participants often work on specific exercises or tasks between seminars.

The management seminars achieve several goals. First, the nursing management staff has a forum for sharing problems and reaping benefits from the expertise of their peers and the administrative staff. Because the managers practice in a variety of areas (for example, inpatient units, operating rooms, ambulatory care units), they have the opportunity to interact with peers whose practice settings are different from their own. They learn that the issues managers face are basically the same in all areas, although the specific incidents may differ. As a result, managers learn to focus on the process for problem solving and can apply the insight a peer brings to their areas. The seminars offer an additional opportunity to interact with and develop a relationship with the administrative staff. Through the seminars, the administrative staff is assured that all nursing management staff has received information about priority issues for the department. Management seminars are an unequaled method of implementing departmentwide change.

In addition, a management forum presented annually should be planned to bring together all managers for a day's worth of content and discussion. The knowledge, skills, and values initiated in seminars are further reinforced in nurse managers' regular meetings with the clinical directors and vice-chairmen.

Phase I. Case Type Analysis Projects

Case type analysis projects are conducted on every inpatient unit by the nursing management staff and have three primary purposes:

1. To analyze the factors that influence length of stay, resource utilization, or both
2. To devise and implement plans to reduce length of stay or resource utilization on the basis of the factors identified
3. To demonstrate the relationship between process, outcome, cost, and length of stay

The projects begin with each unit receiving a computer printout of its most commonly treated DRG categories or case types. From those lists, management staff members of each unit select a study case type in which there are opportunities to reduce resource utilization, length of stay, or both. Next, the management staff is educated about case management plan development and develops a case management plan for the study case type. In the next phase of the project, staff members brainstorm about factors that could be involved in length of stay or resource utilization for the study case type. The factors selected are then entered on the Case Type Analysis Sheet (figure 3-2, see p. 57).

The nurse managers review the literature for pertinent, supportive data. A limited number of patient records are reviewed to verify the effect of the factors identified. The final phase of the project is to develop and implement a plan to reduce length of stay or resource utilization for the study case type.

The study framework is provided by a series of focus questions that are applied to the study case types by the study groups. Those focus questions include the following:

1. What is the nursing product?
2. What is the current nursing production process?
3. What is the time line associated with the production process?
4. What are the factors that influence length of stay and resource utilization?
5. What revisions can be made to the production process that will lower length of stay and cost while achieving satisfactory patient outcomes?
6. How can those revisions be implemented?

The study case type for each unit is then analyzed. Sample findings from NEMCH are summarized in table 3-2 (see pp. 58–59).

Phase II. Implementing Case Management

Case management is a methodology for moving a patient from admission to discharge with outcomes that are determined by quality standards, within a designated time frame, with patient and family participation and control and the astute use and coordination of system resources. After case management is selected as the means of facilitating patient outcomes, the next step is to explore and develop the implications of that methodology.

Implementing case management means developing the methodologies for holding individual primary nurses accountable for patient outcomes. This step requires that a nurse manager's role be formulated with patient/family outcomes, rather than other aspects of care, as the base. The most significant implication is that nurse managers (as the developers of unit-based delivery systems) learn how to measure the results of the components of the production process. All nursing managers and key primary nurses (with a focus on senior staff nurses) are part of this learning process.

The learning objectives for this phase of the management training series are the following:

1. To develop a method for evaluating *individual sets of out-comes* per patient/family per primary nurse
2. To investigate extending the case manager's role beyond unit boundaries
3. To identify a key issue for future research (that is, variables affecting length of stay)

Once the case management model is in place within an institution, the "product" and its "consumer" drive the nursing care delivery system. Costs and pricing are put into a structure that acknowledges the task-completion aspects of professional nursing within the broader context of judgment, advocacy, contracting, and effective management of resources. Because case management plans have put the more complex, multidimensional components of professional nursing practice into a realistic, goal-directed framework, case management can free the geographically bound nurse–patient relationship.

Facilitator Preparation

This section presents recommended curricula for preparing the nurse managers (head nurses) to be facilitators of group practices. The curricula from the monthly management seminars and the facilitation workshop can be expanded or condensed as necessary to fit an institution's unique implementation schedule.

Facilitators of group practices are nurse managers (head nurses) from one of the units prominent for a specific case type. For instance, the head nurse from rehabilitation is a facilitator for the stroke group, whereas the head nurse from the neurology intensive care unit is a facilitator for the craniotomy group. Because the head nurse traditionally has a collaborative relationship with the attending physicians, he or she is in an excellent position to present and negotiate group practice with attending physicians and then to decentralize his or her own authority to the staff nurse case manager. The facilitator spends most of the time coaching the nurse members of the group practice and is occasionally asked to assist at the meetings of the total practice.

The first step in preparing facilitators is to frame the issue as one of decentralizing authority through the teaching of the head nurse's clinical knowledge, collaborative skills, and positive

51

attitudes and values about all aspects of case management. As in implementing all other organizational change at the caregiver level, the head nurse is the person who can make or break it. Head nurses must understand and accept their fundamental role in the design, implementation, and development of case management through group practices. (This role is illustrated in figure 3-3, p. 60). Head nurse facilitators should also attend the three-day curriculum for case managers.

Beyond the management seminar curriculum already presented, it is useful to hold ongoing meetings between facilitators and nursing administrators to offer support and assistance, especially when group practices run into problems that involve several departments. A nursing administrator can suggest effective problem-solving techniques or can take the problem into another arena as necessary. Most problems, however, can be handled by the group practice, and most facilitators are able to help the nursing members meet the objectives outlined in the Group Practice Development Plan (chapter 4).

Once the group practices are off the ground, a one-day workshop for facilitators is in order. The objectives include the following:

1. To list the group practice profile, that is, membership history and data, caseload, patient turnover, length of stay, and so forth, and compare it to that of other practices
2. To identify the stage of development of the group practice
3. To assess each nursing member for his or her ability and performance in case management
4. To determine the next steps to be taken in developing the group practice
5. To evaluate the direction of the group practice in relation to the direction of the institution as a whole

A sample program to meet these objectives is shown in figure 3-4 (see p. 61).

The nurse manager plays a major part in the development of the case manager's role. Including the nurse manager in the educational process of the case manager recognizes the importance of this role while strengthening the nurse manager's understanding of the case management model.

☐ *References*

Gronlund, N. *Stating Objectives for Classroom Instruction*, 2nd ed. New York City: MacMillan Publishing, 1978.

Guy, S., and Comeau, E. *DRGs: A Programmed Instruction*. Boston: Center for Nursing Case Management, New England Medical Center Hospitals, 1986, pp. i–ii.

Loth, R. The no-care zone. *The Boston Globe Magazine*, May 31, 1987.

Peplau, H. Managing toward a professional commitment. In: K. Zander. *Primary Nursing: Development and Management*. Rockville, MD: Aspen Systems Corp., 1980, pp. 53–69.

Peters, T. J. *Thriving on Chaos*. New York City: Alfred A. Knopf, 1987.

Zander, K., and Stetler, C. Case management curriculum. Boston: New England Medical Center Hospitals, developed in 1987.

Table 3-1. 1986 Management Seminars Calendar

Month	Subject	Between Seminar Work
January	Updating case consultation Overview of DRG projects	Review case type analysis projects
February	Measuring health outcomes and complications	Use outcome audit
March	Involving physicians in the case management plans	Meet with physician to develop the CMPs
April	Measuring knowledge outcomes	Use outcome audit
May	Measuring activity (function) outcomes	Use outcome audit
June	Case manager's role: part I	
July	Case manager's role: part II	
August	Analyzing patient acuity/cost	
September	Case manager's role: part III	Report of findings to date, including research questions
October	Anticipating 1987	
November	Measuring the patient/family satisfaction outcomes	Use outcome audit
December	Methodologies for accountability putting it all together	

Source: Copyright, New England Medical Center Hospitals, 1987.

Figure 3-1. 1987 Management Seminars: "Directions in Case Management"

Objectives

1. Identify key skills and structures essential to the case manager's role.

2. Formulate management approaches that support the implementation of case management beyond the senior staff level.

3. Evaluate the implementation of the case management role for a specific case type, collaborative practice, and unit.

Month	Content
January	Vertical teams: Management forum HMO contracts/managed care Preliminary findings from case management diaries From case management plans to critical paths
February	Assessment: Functional assessment Family assessment Case manager consultation
March	Formal collaborative practices: Formation Negotiation Authority Consultation Case manager consultation
April	From assessment to goals: Nursing diagnosis Goal setting Contracting Case manager consultation
May	Monitoring progress and resources: Critical paths Use of rounds Case manager consultation
June	Evaluating case managers: Case manager consultation
July	Educating for self-care, self-medication: Case manager consultation
August	Use of the telephone: Case manager consultation

Continued on next page

Figure 3-1. (Continued)

Month	Content
September	Working with the health care team: Case manager consultation
October	Home health care: Case manager consultation
November	Identifying case manager learning needs: Case manager consultation
December	Evaluating outcomes objectively: Toward peer audit

Source: Copyright, New England Medical Center Hospitals, 1987.

Figure 3-2. Case Type Analysis Sheet

Diagnosis _____   Length of Stay _____

Unit _____   MDC _____

DRG _____   Usual OR Day _____

Patient	LOS	Age	Sex	PN	MD				

Table 3-2. Summary of Sample Case Type Analysis Projects

Case Type	Unit	Reported by	Goals	Examples of Factors Studied	Methodology for Reducing Length of Stay/Resources
Coronary artery bypass graft	Cardiothoracic intensive care	Donna Wood	Reduce ICU stay by 12–24 hours	• Smoking history • Arrhythmias • Preop patient unit • Number of MIs • Arrhythmias • Severity of coronary artery disease • Amount of preop teaching • Preop medications • Baseline vital signs	• Utilization of transfer information sheet developed by nurse managers of CTU and preop cardiac surgery units • Preop teaching on cardiac surgical unit
Laparoscopy	Day surgery center	Patricia Kavanaris	Reduce unplanned admissions after day surgery	• Preop patient screening • Postop nausea and vomiting • Pain management	• Development of a new pre/postop patient record, including patient teaching • Utilization of intraoperative antiemetics • Development of written postoperative handout
Abdominal aortic aneurysm	Surgical intensive care unit	Winifred Walker	Reduce ICU length of stay	• Primary nurse experience level • Presence of renal or respiratory conditions • Smoking history • Patient anxiety level	• Utilization of case management plan to educate new primary nurses • Implementation of a new AAA teaching plan emphasizing the need to stop smoking preoperatively and postop pulmonary care

Primary total hip replacement (THR)	Orthopedics	Michell Small Judith Cronin	Reduce length of stay		
				• Age • Past medical and surgical history • PT visit preop • PT visit postop and frequency of visits • Patient compliance • Functional baseline activity level • Family supports • Social Service involvement • When discharge planning began	• Primary nurses educated about placement procedures and availability of external resources • Early contact with PT • Efficient RN-MD collaboration about discharge planning through daily rounds and communication with Social Service • Placement of the patient within two days of clearance • Number of transfers to the hospital's rehabilitation unit increased • Early discussions initiated with patient and family by primary nurse regarding discharge plans considering baseline functioning and available supports • Expanded involvement of support services in discharge rounds

Source: Copyright, New England Medical Center Hospitals, 1987.

Figure 3-3.   Role of Nurse Managers to Support Case Management

1. Continue to maintain the primary nursing system on the unit

2. Maintain managed care for all patients on the unit by using critical paths as the basis of report

3. Develop unit/group practice management tools, roles, and methods for feedback about cost/quality outcomes; for example, CMPs, CPs, audits, and so forth, and collaborate in development of related departmental standards

4. Implement initial group practices by
   - Introducing concept to attending physicians
   - Selecting nurse(s) from your unit through planning with clinical director and other nurse managers
   - Introducing nurse members to attending physicians
   - Sending nurses to case management curriculum

5. Maintain group practices
   - Interview and appoint new members, using input from current members and the attending physicians
   - Meet weekly with the nursing members from your unit to review the patient roster
   - As much as possible, accommodate attendance at regular and unscheduled group practice meetings
   - Facilitate development of knowledge base of group members and provide appropriate resources/opportunities
   - Establish a regular pattern of communication with attending physicians to discuss case management issues
   - Act as an ad hoc consultant for case consultation sessions
   - Evaluate nursing members of the practice from annual basis using the new form, which will include input from a variety of sources (audits, peer review, anecdotes, and so forth)

6. Further develop case management
   - Meet monthly with the nursing members of the group practice to review their management plan and progress toward quarterly goals
   - Assist in the formal evaluation of the case management model
   - Meet regularly with other nurse managers from related group practices to review progress and needs

Figure 3-4. Sample Program for One-Day Facilitators' Workshop

A. Collaborative practice profile

   Membership
   History
   Data

B. Case management update

   Catastrophic illness
   Changes in the health care industry as they relate to the institution
   Changes in the institution as they relate to group practices

C. Development of group practices

   Evaluation of individual members
   Group dynamics and group growth (theory)
   Evaluation of members collectively

D. Methods to stabilize and foster group practices

   Post implementation
   Membership issues
   Communication issues
   Coordination issues
   Continuity issues
   Case consultation
   Outcome measurement
   Clinical questions
   Financial feedback

Implementing Nursing Case Management

The implementation of case management is undertaken after the initial process, outcome, and time standards have been established for target case types and after the key physicians and nurses have been identified and educated. In fact, implementation marks the end of perhaps the most complex phase of case management and the beginning of the most rewarding phase for everyone. If the preparation work of design, education, and team building has been solid, then each group practice will have the foundation upon which to implement case-specific management. Certain approaches have proved useful. All the approaches undergo revision as the practice of case management evolves. As suggested by Zander (1988, p. 24):

> There is nothing easy or magical about building a model for case management, except perhaps the energy that is rechanneled from struggling with chronic bureaucratic situations to real solutions for patient-centered care. It requires administration's relentless focus, openness, and risk-taking, all difficult approaches to keep while maintaining the usual operations of a department.

☐ Ground Rules for Case Management

Although each group practice is independent in its clinical decision making, it is interdependent with other elements within the larger institution. Therefore, institutionwide ground rules are helpful in the implementation and evaluation phases. The following ground rules can be applied by beginning with one or two physicians and case types at a time (revised from Twyon, 1987):

1. Every designated patient is admitted to a formally prepared group practice composed of an attending physician and a specific group practice of staff nurses from each of the units and clinics likely to receive those patients.
2. All nurses in the group practice give direct care as the patient's primary or associate nurse while the patient is on his or her geographic unit.
3. Every group practice assigns one of its nursing members to be the case manager who works with the attending physician in evaluating an individualized case management plan (CMP) and critical path (CP) for each patient.
4. A critical path for the whole episode of care is used to manage the care of every designated patient, both at change of shift report and during group practice meetings.
5. Nursing members of the group practice meet on a weekly basis at a consistent time and place and maintain a patient roster.
6. Each member of the group practice communicates immediate patient care issues with the attending physician while the patient is on his or her own unit. The assigned case manager works through the group and the attending for nonemergency issues.
7. Negative variances from critical paths or CMPs require discussion with the attending physician and a case management consultation when necessary.
8. The group practice meets to discuss care patterns, policies, specific patients and variances, and research questions and to update knowledge at their own predetermined intervals, for example, monthly or bimonthly. Minutes are taken for reference by members who cannot attend.
9. Group practice members negotiate a flexible schedule that accommodates the needs of their case-managed patients and group practices, as well as the needs of their units.
10. The responsibility of the case manager begins with a notification of the patient's entry into the system and

ends with a formal transfer of accountability to the patient, the patient's family, another health care provider, or another institution.

☐ Management Tools and Systems

In addition to case management plans and critical paths, tools and systems for managing cases with group practices emerge as the clinicians and administrators see the need. Some generic tools and systems are the following:

- A patient roster, kept in a notebook at a location central to the group practice (figure 4-1, see p. 83)
- A system for notifying the group practice about when patients are going to be admitted (as in surgery) or have been admitted (as in emergencies) (this system often involves the attending physician's secretary, the attending physician, the operating room scheduling staff, or the emergency room member of a group practice)
- An introductory letter and group practice business card sent to scheduled patients (figures 4-2 and 4-3, see pp. 84–85)
- A folder or portfolio in which patients and families can keep written information and their copy of the critical path throughout the episode of illness

Obviously, computerized medical records and other sophisticated tracking and information systems only enhance the abilities of clinicians to manage their cases across an episode of illness and throughout an institution. Case management, however, depends more on person-to-person communication than on high-tech tools. The addition of another telephone line may be more valuable to clinicians than more expensive items.

☐ Group Practice Development Plan: Postcurriculum

The group practices are a continuation of the team building instituted as part of the case management curriculum. After group development work is under way, the group practice can address the clinical issues it was formed to tackle. A sample group practice development plan is shown in figure 4-4 (see pp. 86–89).

☐ Meetings and Facilitators

One of the key operational ground rules is that the group practice nurses meet on a weekly basis and that the whole group practice, including physicians, meets at regular intervals. These meetings serve to forge vital links among caregivers as well as to perform the important function of reviewing policies and patterns of care for groups of case type–specific patients.

The meetings of group practice nurses are held weekly for no longer than an hour: same place, same day, same time every week. This structure allows staff nurses to arrange their schedules. It also enables their nurse managers (head nurses) to ensure coverage for on-unit activities and responsibilities. Overtime is not used for this coverage, and nurses are not expected to come to meetings on their days off or while they are on vacation.

In the first year, it is useful to have a nurse manager from one of the units represented in the group practice act as a facilitator for the group. The initial facilitation involves assisting the group with its development plan (see the discussion of preparation for nurse managers in chapter 3). The purpose of much of the facilitation work is to develop the group's creative problem-solving skills. Because of their familiarity with the larger institution, nurse managers at times have access to people and information formerly out of a staff nurse's domain, and they can offer system-savvy knowledge to the group.

Thus, the head nurse is facilitator, teacher, and coach. He or she suggests collaborative approaches, stimulates inquiry into the status quo, expects clinical and financial outcomes to be addressed, and offers problem-solving expertise.

Meetings with the nurses and attending physician(s) are not necessary for the daily and weekly monitoring of all cases, but they are useful for periodic review and evaluation of the care of groups of patients. In these meetings, larger system issues are identified, new clinical information is shared, and new ideas can be explored. A facilitator might be present if deemed useful by the group practice.

Collaborative practice at the caregiver level is a more practical and acceptable expenditure of time than joint practice committees that strive for the same overall results but quickly lose momentum. Physicians and nurses do care about cost and quality issues, and they should be willing to be involved in this immediately meaningful work.

☐ Organizational Development Plan

As new group practices are formed and the current ones begin to suggest changes that may affect other departments and systems, certain individuals must be responsive to them. These individuals may be different in each institution, but should include top hospital administrators, including the chairman of nursing and the physician chiefs.

Organizational development, that is, planned change from the top down, becomes a necessity as the institution increasingly commits itself to case management. Eventually, case management will affect all of the institution's systems. Some of the first to be affected are:

- Admitting
- Documentation/medical records
- Laboratories and pharmacy
- Discharge planning/continuing care
- Cost per case/acuity/utilization data collection

The two most important aspects in developing a case management model are (1) to collect baseline data of costs and quality per case type before implementation and (2) to mutually agree on realistic cost and quality outcomes that might occur as a result of case management. After these two steps, a strategic plan should take about two months to develop, followed by education of head nurses and education of group practices. The whole process will be strengthened if managed care and primary nursing have already been implemented.

In summary, the development of case management is an evolving, dynamic process. It requires a foundation of expert planning and design and, most important, a constant responsiveness to the clinicians, their needs, and their results.

☐ Tools of Implementation: Case Management Plans

The operation of a case management model calls for the development and use of specific strategies and tools. The focus of this section is a tool called *case management plans*. Their purpose, structure, and evolution will be described next, as well as issues pertinent to potential users.

The Purpose and Function of CMPs

Case management plans (or CMPs) are time-lined, standardized plans of care for patients in a specific diagnostic case type. Each plan consists of the following components:

- Nursing-related problems
- Patient outcomes
- Patient intermediate outcomes
- Nursing interventions
- Physician interventions
- Target times

An excerpt from a CMP for the case type diagnosis of stroke is provided in figure 4-5 (see pp. 90–93). Target times (that is, hour, day, or week) are specified in relation to the patient's projected length of stay. Furthermore, the plan's content is expected to reflect current practice, resource use, and status of the majority (75 to 100 percent) of patients within the case type, across the entire episode of illness. A plan, therefore, probably consists of multiple subsections representative of the patient care units through which the patient progresses during the course of the illness treatment. For example, the stroke CMP consists of the following sections in this order: emergency department, neurology intensive care unit, general neurology unit, rehabilitation unit, and ambulatory neurology clinic.

In some respects, CMPs are similar to the general concept of a generic or standardized nursing care plan. However, their purpose and focus within the framework of case management are somewhat different. More specifically:

1. CMPs provide an explicit description of the product currently provided to a specific case type. *Product* is defined as both a service and an expected patient outcome. Concomitantly, these two factors allow for a review of targets of opportunity for the improvement of the cost-effectiveness of care delivery, that is, for product improvement.
2. CMPs provide a mechanism for the explicit review of interdisciplinary function in relation to the care of a specific case type and, thereby, for validation of nursing's scope of practice and expectations for collaborative interaction. Although only the activities of physicians and

nurses are incorporated into the examples provided, columns for additional professionals may be added.

3. CMPs make explicit the focus of nursing care and thus serve as an educational tool for both nurses and other care providers. They also clarify the need to address the continuity and consistency of care across both units and care providers.

Case management plans were first developed at the New England Medical Center Hospitals to "define the business of nursing as the essential link between tasks and clinical outcomes" (DeZell, 1987, p. 4) (figure 4-6, see p. 94). However, when the tool was viewed in relation to an overall model of care delivery, it became increasingly obvious that professional practice is now a collective enterprise. Nursing care, as indicated by the nature of the identified problems, continues to be the primary focus of case management plans. However, recognition of the related responsibilities of physicians, as well as of the need for their support of nursing's critical role in the care process, is essential in implementing true collaborative practice and, thus, in the delivery of the most cost-effective care possible. It is vital, therefore, to share CMPs with key attending physicians to obtain their input and support, as well as to identify related physician interventions.

The patient is also a part of this collective enterprise. Intermediate outcomes, which are defined as progressive steps or indicators displayed by the patient (or family) that provide evidence regarding movement toward defined outcomes (Stetler and DeZell, 1987), clearly indicate patient involvement and responsibility.

Standardization

Once the initial purpose and format are established, case management plans can be developed. A standardized framework or terminology is strongly recommended at the outset in order to achieve the following goals:

- CMPs can be easily understood by nurses on the unit of origin and throughout the department of nursing (as well as in the general nursing community).
- Computerization can be implemented.
- Research can be conducted on any aspect of the CMPs.

At New England Medical Center Hospitals, a task force was created for the purpose of standardizing the content of case management plans. Members of the task force included nurse managers, staff nurses, senior staff nurses, a supervisor, and a staff educator. The group was cochaired by the nurse researcher and the projects coordinator.

The following approach to the standardization process was found to be feasible:

1. A standard list of problems for use as a reference tool for nurses formulating or revising CMPs was developed.
2. A model set of outcomes (both intermediate and final) was developed to illustrate, per problem, the expected progression and thereby allow for concurrent evaluation of a problem's resolution.
3. Nurses were provided with reference manuals that further describe the accepted list of problems within a nursing diagnostic framework (for example, definition-defining characteristics).

The following summary, based on the experience of New England Medical Center Hospitals in developing more than 130 case management plans, is offered as a further guideline to the process.

Standard Problem List

In order to avoid reinventing the wheel, the task force consulted multiple resources. In general, the approved nomenclature of the National Conference on the Classification of Nursing Diagnoses (or NANDA list) is a good starting point (Hurley, 1986; Kim and others, 1984; McLane, 1987). However, the following questions must be answered by the task force early in the development process:

- Must nursing diagnoses (that is, nursing-related "problems") solely reflect independence of action, particularly in light of the collaborative nature of the case management model?
- Does the current NANDA list sufficiently reflect acute care nursing?
- Do certain widely used diagnoses accurately define the true nature of a patient's problem and the desired outcome of patient care?

"Knowledge deficit" is the most critical example of the third question and is thus deliberately excluded from the standard problem list developed by New England Medical Center Hospitals task force. "Lack of knowledge" is believed to more accurately reflect a risk factor or etiology because the primary focus is to prevent complications, not to provide knowledge in and of itself; Jenny (1987) presents a similar argument.

Another major difference between the New England Medical Center Hospitals task force's standard list and the NANDA list is the development or redefinition of four diagnoses:

1. Potential for injury/complication unrelated to treatment
2. Potential for complication related to treatment
3. Potential for extension of the disease process
4. Potential for complication/self-care

Each of these diagnoses in reality represents a general category of problem and requires a clarifying subcategory; for example, "potential for complication/self-care" has, as a subcategory, "inappropriate administration of medication." Each of the four diagnoses, however, provides an explicit reason or name for many of the activities in which nurses engage in an acute care setting. These activities are nursing, not medical, although some are interdependent; and their focus is the prevention of deleterious responses to treatment or the environment, or the prevention of further deterioration of an unhealthful state, within the limits of medical technology and the disease process.

Each of these diagnoses is described in figures 4-7 through 4-10 (see pp. 95–98). Of note, however, are the following:

1. These problems provide a means to eliminate the use of "medical" diagnoses from case management plans, which nurses so frequently resort to because of a lack of appropriate terminology. In particular, this is true for the diagnosis "potential for extension of the disease process." Although the clarifying subcategory is usually a medical diagnosis or symptom that also requires major medical attention, the problem category itself refocuses the purpose of the intervention to nursing's realm. The University Hospitals of Cleveland (1986) have a nursing diagnosis (that is, instability) with an intent that appears similar. Two other nursing diagnoses of related note are:

    a. High risk of secondary brain injury (Joint Committee to Revise Standards of Neuroscience Nursing Practice, 1985, p. 5)

    b. Potential complication: Cardiac arrhythmias related to hypokalemia (ANA and Oncology Nursing Society, 1987, p. 24)

2. Along with potential diagnoses from NANDA, these problems provide a clear picture of the significant amount of nursing time that is devoted to prevention of nursing, medical, and patient-dependent complications.

3. The diagnosis of "potential for complication/self-care" makes the preparation of patients for discharge an explicit and distinctly important problem. The clarifying sub-categories, which can be multiple, help to focus the nurse on the reason for providing knowledge, skill, and support to patients and their families and, simultaneously, focus the nurse on the outcomes to be achieved, not on an interim step such as verbalization of understanding.

Listed below are examples of the problems that are expected to occur in most patients in two case types. From the listing, it is clear that nursing care is essential to the well-being of these individuals.

Case type: Adult leukemia (inpatient, general medical unit)
- Anxiety
- Grieving
- Activity intolerance (fatigue)
- Nutrition, less than body requirements
- Alteration in oral mucous membrane
- Potential for infection
- Potential for bleeding
- Potential for complications related to treatment, that is, adverse medication side effects
- Potential for fluid volume deficit
- Potential for complication/self-care
  - Infection
  - Bleeding
  - Activity intolerance
  - Nutrition, less than body requirements
  - Inappropriate medication administration, adverse side effects, or both

Case type: Uncomplicated myocardial infarction (ambulatory)
- Pain
- Potential for decreased cardiac output
- Anxiety
- Potential for complication/self-care
  - Medication side effects
  - Extension of the disease process (for example, myocardial infarction/angina)

In developing a case management plan for case types such as adult leukemia and myocardial infarction, the focus is on those problems that are *critical to the case type.* To keep CMPs at a reasonable length, care generic to broader categories of patients (for example, surgical or medical) is not included in specific detail. Instead, a special notation is made at the end of each CMP entitled "additional potential problems/complications," and under this heading routine concerns and activities are briefly listed. This mechanism is particularly valuable in that the tools can also be used for orientation of new nurses who might not have knowledge of generic standards. For example, the following potential problems/complications are addressed under this heading on the uncomplicated myocardial infarction CMP developed by the inpatient adult general medical unit:

- Peripheral line infection
- Constipation
- Impairment of skin integrity
- Embolus formation
- Ineffective airway clearance

Finally, although a number of references were used in developing the standard list, one in particular should be noted: *Applied Nursing Diagnosis* by K. Gettrust, S. Ryan, and D. S. Engleman (1985). Its practical approach and extensive content are extremely useful; and its value can perhaps best be measured by the continuous disappearance of copies from the committee as nurses took them to use on the units as a routine reference. (For a list of the multiple sources used in the work on CMPs, see the reference list at the end of this chapter.)

Standardized Outcome Index

The nursing literature frequently cites the importance of patient outcomes or various approaches to their evaluation within the service setting (Gallant and McLane, 1979; Hover and Zimmer, 1978; Inzer and Aspinal, 1981; Luker, 1981; Marker, 1988; Osinski, 1987; Westfall, 1986). However, no extensive list of outcomes made on the basis of nursing outcomes was found that allows easy measurability on a routine basis in the acute care setting and concisely defines outcomes in light of a progressive set of intermediate indicators in relation to the final resolution or prevention of a problem. Horn and Swain's work (1978) is valuable as a resource, but it is not directly based on a nursing diagnostic framework nor is it a concise, progressive tool. Gettrust and others (1985) provide a valuable reference, but they merge intermediate and final outcomes. They also, understandably, provide a wide variety of outcome possibilities rather than one model set of critical outcomes per problem.

The New England Medical Center Hospitals task force concluded that a sample or index of outcomes is needed. This index should clearly and concisely outline for the nurse a possible means of concurrently evaluating a patient's progress relative to resolution or prevention of each nursing problem on the standard list. The model must present critical progressive indicators, not an exhaustive list, and it must be user friendly, that is, useful for documentation and capable of being easily modified to adapt to the individual status of a patient.

On the basis of multiple resources (for example, Bufalino and Caine, 1987; Crosley and others, 1985; Doenges and others, 1984; Gluck, 1975; Westfall, 1986), the following five-step process for development of the final index was eventually developed:

1. Develop a preliminary draft of progressive outcome indicators for a specified number of problems by an assigned subgroup of panel members. Reference material must be cited.
2. Review and revise the preliminary draft by a second subgroup of panel members. One member of the initial subgroup should be included.
3. Review resulting outcomes by the task force as a whole. Emphasis should be placed on the following:

- The relevance of the draft outcomes to current case management plans
- Clarity and appropriateness of the progression of indicators as well as of the critical nature of the included outcomes
- Final consensus for all draft components
4. Arrange for review by in-house nursing experts or units where drafted problems frequently occur, with:
   - Several panel members assigned per problem
   - Experts/units asked to review draft and then pilot test on actual patients
5. Prepare final revision based on feedback from nursing experts/units.

Once developed for each problem on the standardized problem list, the generic set of progressive outcomes is included in the CMPs, thus creating a standardized outcome list per individual case type. The set of model outcomes is adapted to the degree necessary for each case type and individual. This is accomplished through the identification/statement of specific measurement parameters appropriate to the individual/case type. In the end, the standardized outcome list will provide a ready means of monitoring the progress of a patient through explicit outcome criteria that are clear to all care providers and that are framed within the concept of length of stay.

Issues in CMP Development and Use

Developing CMPs by case type is a critical step in the evolution/ implementation of the nursing case management model. These collaborative plans lay the groundwork for stronger formal relationships, group practices, and clinical contracts between nurses and physicians as the central providers of patient care (DeZell, 1987).

As the CMPs are revised using the standardized list of problems, standard outcomes (as available), and relevant reference material, their clarity and nursing focus are enhanced. However, their length may be considerably increased. Length is not a consideration when the tool is viewed as an orientation strategy for new graduates or experienced nurses unfamiliar with a given case type. Length should also not be a consideration when separate sections of the plan are used as a mechanism to review continuity of care. Viewed in its entirety, the complete plan can be used to assess redundancies or inconsistencies across the total episode of illness and care providers.

Length *is* critical, however, when one views CMPs in relation to day-to-day evaluation and documentation.

As such, in the absence of computerization, CMPs are not practical for use on a day-to-day basis as a permanent manual documentation tool; that is, handwritten modification through an individual patient's needs and charting of the patient care provided are difficult. Yet the overall value of CMPs relative to product identification, interdisciplinary function, and education remains.

Therefore, to facilitate the goals of case management until computerization, the following steps should be taken:

1. Develop critical paths, which are one-page, user-friendly tools derived from case management plans that focus primarily on the key tasks or technical aspects of care that must be completed within a specified time frame if cost-effective care is to be achieved. These tools are easily kept in the patient kardex to continually reinforce the importance of coordinating and tracking the critical components of care. (Critical paths are more fully discussed later in this chapter.)
2. As case management plans are revised, develop standardized case type packets that include the case management plan, the critical path, and the existing permanent documentation tools (nursing index and treatment sheets) that have been completed with the appropriate data excerpted from the case management plans (that is, patient problems and outcomes, nursing interventions).

These are effective measures in the short run, until computerization and on-line documentation are accomplished. Institutions with computerization in place should be able to efficiently utilize the case management plan and critical paths in their current format. Computerization is a far superior approach because, as fully integrated operative tools, case management plans document the link between process and outcomes at the clinical level and emphasize the nursing process as the essence of professional nursing practice.

Two final comments are in order. First, it must be made clear that case management plans are general guidelines for the care of the majority of patients within a designated case type. They are not absolute standards and must be used by clinicians with sufficient knowledge to adapt them to the unique needs of individual patients. Second, development of CMPs should ideally be based on a body of research. This is a difficult task, given the stage of development of nursing diagnoses and the time required. As currently developed at New England Medical Center Hospitals, case management plans, as well as critical paths and standardized outcome indexes, are made primarily on the basis of the clinical knowledge of experienced nurses supplemented by pertinent resources from the literature and, in selected cases, review by the task force. This is a valuable base and, in terms of time, an efficient one. For the future, it is recognized that both the use of current research findings and the conduct of research could enhance the validity of all of these tools. Involvement of graduate students and funding requests are two strategies to increase the integration of research into this valuable process.

□ Tools of Implementation: Critical Paths

Efforts to control escalating health care costs have resulted in shorter hospital stays and increased acuity of hospitalized patients with greater support needs upon discharge. A timely and appropriate diagnostic evaluation and treatment plan, as well as care in an appropriate setting, become important considerations in containing costs. At the same time, early identification of discharge dates and attention to discharge planning become critical to prepare the patient who requires home care services and to ensure the appropriate use of hospital beds.

Hospitals are asking clinicians not only to make their patients well but to do so in the most cost-effective manner, that is, within a designated or appropriate length of stay, using appropriate resources. Eliminating the first and last days of hospitalization, at first glance, seems like an easy way to reduce length of stay. But once done, what happens next? To answer this question, clinicians must examine what happens to a given case type on each day of hospitalization.

Answering some of the following key questions provides a framework for plotting the course of hospitalization for a given case type. For instance, when does the admission diagnostic workup occur, on day 1 or day 2 of admission? What is included in the workup? When do key consultations take place? When must tests be ordered so that they are completed in a timely fashion? When should teaching be initiated so that appropriate behaviors are learned before discharge? When does the nasogastric tube come out? When does ambulation start? When is a full diet resumed? All of these factors plus many more often significantly influence the length of stay.

In searching for a way to make this process more tangible so that it can be visualized and evaluated, a tool called *critical paths* was developed for each major case type. Critical paths are abbreviated versions of case management plans. They show the critical or key incidents that must occur in a predictable and timely fashion to achieve an appropriate length of stay. The key incidents of a critical path are categorized according to consultations, diagnostic tests, activities, treatments, diet, medications, discharge planning, and teaching (figure 4-11, see pp. 99–100).

Development

A primary nurse and attending physician who work primarily with a given case type develop a standard critical path for that case type (for example, myocardial infarction, unstable angina, cholecystectomy). This is done by outlining the key incidents that must occur for the specific case type while simultaneously considering the time frames that need to be followed to meet length-of-stay parameters and to control resource utilization.

Utilization

Within 24 hours of the patient's admission to the hospital, the primary nurse and physician develop an individualized critical path for the patient, taking into consideration comorbidities and socioeconomic factors. If changes from the standard are to be made, they are identified at this time. From this point on, all deviations from the critical path are considered variances. These variances are identified on a daily basis and put into three categories of causality: caused by something within the patient, caused by the system, or caused by the caregivers. The variances are either justified by the primary nurse and attending physician or actions are immediately taken to rectify the variance.

Daily Use

Critical paths are reviewed by the nursing staff during intershift report, three times per day. Intershift report includes information on expected length of stay, critical incidents that should occur that day, and variances from the standard. If variances occur, a consultation with the primary nurse's peers is conducted immediately after report. The critical paths are also used on attending physicians' and house officers' rounds.

Other Uses

Initially, critical paths were developed to be used directly with patients. Since then, several other equally important applications have been found.

Orientation of Nurses and House Staff

One case manager commented to a visiting physician that the critical paths enabled new clinicians to understand the total process of care. She went on to explain that what had taken her two years to learn and understand through constant experience with a case type could be mastered by a clinician within six weeks.

Physicians and nurses are taught pathophysiology and the treatment of disease. However, they are never taught, either in schools or in orientation to new jobs, how to institute and carry out a treatment plan in the most cost-effective and timely manner. Using the critical paths, new clinicians have easy access to information regarding usual length of stay and the key incidents that must be attended to. Even the inexperienced clinician can identify variances quickly. In a sense, critical paths put new clinicians in control by giving them a tool to assist in planning with the attending physician and to help them communicate the plan of care to patients and their families.

Changing Practice

Critical paths are extremely useful in helping clinicians identify targets of opportunity to alter the usual treatment plan for a given case type. Critical paths help clinicians clearly visualize current practice and indicate when either nothing is being done for the patient or too much is being done.

In developing a critical path for patients undergoing induction therapy for leukemia, for example, the usual practice was to admit the patient two to four days before putting in a Cooks catheter. Chemotherapy was then started, followed by antibiotic therapy, antifungal therapy, or both, and continued for three to four weeks. A complete fever workup was done at least once a day. Electrolyte values and a complete blood count were also determined daily. Reviewing subsequent readmissions revealed that the patient was hospitalized four more times for consolidation treatment with chemotherapy.

After examining current practice, the following changes were made: (1) the Cooks catheter is placed in the patient on day 2 of hospitalization; (2) when the patient is no longer neutropenic and is afebrile, antibiotic therapy and antifungal therapy are completed at home; (3) mouth care for thrush is begun on day 1, before symptoms are evident; (4) if no new organism is identified, a fever workup is done every 48 hours; and (5) only essential electrolyte values and blood counts are determined on a daily basis. These changes have reduced the patient's length of stay from six to eight weeks (42–56 days) to approximately four weeks (32 days). Unnecessary diagnostic tests have been eliminated. Low-dose consolidation chemotherapy is now being given at home, thus eliminating 14 additional days of hospitalization. By implementing these changes, quality outcomes were not only maintained but improved. Infection rates decreased with home chemotherapy; patients slept through the night when a complete fever workup was not done; much more time was spent at home with families; and finally, patients reported increased satisfaction with care and a feeling that they were in better control of what happened to them. The use of critical paths has established three main points:

1. Surgical case types are much more predictable and more likely to follow a standard critical path than are medical case types.

2. Medical case types often have other problems during hospitalization that necessitate superimposed critical. paths; for example, unstable angina may become myocardial infarction, or the patient may also require angioplasty.
3. Adjustment of the standard must always be considered to include comorbidities and psychosocial issues.

Clinicians' Response

In summary, a comment should be made on how critical paths have been received by clinicians. Nurses and doctors find them easy to develop because the process simply requires them to outline their work. Physicians welcome them as a way to ensure that what they want for their patients is done in a timely fashion. Administrators, finance officers, and third-party payers view them as concrete evidence that clinicians are actively addressing the most efficient ways to care for patients while maintaining quality. Finally, critical paths empower nurses to feel more in control of the treatment plan and more effective as collaborators with the physician.

□ *References and Bibliography*

American Nurses' Association and Oncology Nursing Society. *Standards of Oncology Nursing Practice.* Kansas City, MO: ANA, 1987.

Bufalino, P., and Caine, R. *Nursing Care Planning Guides for Adults.* Baltimore: Williams & Wilkins, 1987.

Crosley, J., Bizzard, C., Brooks, C., Fink, L., Foegl, R., Graison-Smith, B., Molloy, D., and O'Brien, J. *Computerized Nursing Care Planning Utilizing Nursing Diagnoses: A Handbook.* Washington, DC: Oryn Publications, 1985.

DeZell, A. D. Case management plans: a collaborative model. *Definition* 2(1):1–4, 1987.

Doenges, M. E., Jeffries, and Moorehouse. *Nursing Care Plans: Nursing Diagnoses in Planning Patient Care.* Philadelphia: F. A. Davis, 1984.

Gallant, B., and McLane, A. Outcome criteria: a process for validation at the unit level. *Journal of Nursing Administration* 9(1):14–21, 1979.

Gettrust, K., Ryan, S., and Engleman, D. *Applied Nursing Diagnosis: Guides for Comprehensive Care Planning.* New York City: John Wiley & Sons, 1985.

Gluck, J. Clinical nurse specialist in pulmonary medicine: a prospectus. Unpublished paper, Boston University School of Nursing, Boston, no date. [Cited in Zander, K. *Primary Nursing: Development and Management.* Rockville, MD: Aspen Systems Corp., 1975.]

Horn, B., and Swain, M. *Manual for Instrument of Health Status Measures.* Vol. II, *Development of Criterion Measures of Nursing Care* (NTIS no. PB 267005). Springfield, VA: National Technical Information Service, 1978.

Hover, J., and Zimmer, M. Nursing quality assurance: the Wisconsin system. *Nursing Outlook* 26(4):242–48, 1978.

Hurley, M., editor. *Classification of Nursing Diagnoses: Proceedings of the Sixth Conference.* St. Louis: C. V. Mosby, 1986.

Inzer, F., and Aspinal, M. Evaluating patient outcomes. *Nursing Outlook* 29(3):178–81, 1981.

Jenny, J. Knowledge deficit: not a nursing diagnosis. *Image: Journal of Nursing Scholarship* 19:184–85, 1987.

Joint Committee to Revise Standards of Neuroscience Nursing Practice. *Neuroscience Nursing Practice: Process and Outcome Criteria for Selected Diagnoses.* Kansas City, MO: American Nurses' Association, 1985.

Kim, M., McFarland, G., and McLane, H., editors. *Classification of Nursing Diagnoses: Proceedings of the Fifth Conference.* St. Louis: C. V. Mosby, 1984.

Luker, K. An overview of evaluation research in nursing. *Journal of Advanced Nursing* 6(2):87–93, 1981.

Marker, C. G. Smith. Practical tools for quality assurance: criteria development sheet and data retrieval form. *Journal of Nursing Quality Assurance* 2:43–54, 1988.

McLane, A., editor. *Classification of Nursing Diagnoses: Proceedings of the Seventh Conference.* St. Louis: C. V. Mosby, 1987.

Osinski, E. Developing patient outcomes as a quality measure of nursing care. *Nursing Management* 18:28–29, 1987.

Stetler, C., and DeZell, A. D. *Case Management Plans: Designs for Transformation.* Boston: Center for Nursing Case Management, New England Medical Center Hospitals, 1987.

Twyon, S. *Ground Rules: Case Management.* Boston: New England Medical Center Hospitals, 1987.

University Hospitals of Cleveland. Unpublished memo, 1986.

Westfall, U. Outcome criteria generation: a process and product. In: M. Hurley, editor. *Classification of Nursing Diagnoses: Proceedings of the Sixth Conference.* St. Louis: C. V. Mosby, 1986.

Zander, K. Nursing case management: strategic management of cost and quality outcomes. *Journal of Nursing Administration* 18(5):24, May 1988.

Figure 4-1. Group Practice Patient Roster

Group Practice: _____   Date: _____

Patient's Name	Admit Date	Date Case Manager Assigned	Case Manager	Diagnosis	Standard LOS*	Revised LOS**	Actual Input D/C Date	Date Critical Path Initiated	Date D/C from Coll. Practice

*List the expected length of stay as listed on the *standard* critical path.

**If the expected length of stay was changed for the patient from the standard *within the first 24 hours* of admission due to comorbidities, list the revised length of stay here.

Source: Copyright, New England Medical Center Hospitals, 1987.

Figure 4-2. Introductory Letter

Dear _____.

As a nurse who works at New England Medical Center Hospitals, I would like to introduce myself as a member of the Neurosurgery Collaborative Practice. I work with Dr. Shucart and his patients who are admitted for surgery. I will be contacting you by telephone before your admission, at which time we can discuss your expected hospital course. This will be a good opportunity for you to ask questions regarding your nursing care.

Sincerely,

_____
Your case manager

Figure 4-3. Group Practice Business Card (Front and Back)

Neurosurgery Collaborative Practice
Carol-Jane G. Albertelli, RN
ICU ext. 5808
Lynn Costello, RN
Inpatient ext. 5805
Janet Parker, RN
Rehabilitation ext. 5639
William Shucart, MD
Office ext. 5858

Case Manager _____

New England
Medical Center Hospitals

750 Washington Street
Boston, MA 02111
Telephone (617) 956-5000

Your case manager is a primary nurse who works with you, your family, and the health care team to coordinate your care in the hospital and after discharge. Your case manager is a member of a collaborative practice that includes your physician and selected inpatient and outpatient nurses.

Figure 4-4. Group Practice Development Plan

Group Practice Name: _____   Facilitator: _____

Objectives	Activities	Staff	Target Date	Progress Reports
1. Complete creation of an initial case management packet for group members	i. Integrate the critical path across total episode of illness ii. Collect all relevant teaching materials iii. Collect and read case-related literature iv. Review standardized case management plans (as available) for total episode v. Other: for example, • Protocols • Flow sheets			
2. Establish/identify systems of communication among group members	i. Establish a meeting time and location ii. Establish a system for communicating with absent members iii. Establish a system for communicating with attending physician(s): • Who will initially approach the attending physician(s)? • What will be communicated? iv. Agree upon the method for maintaining ongoing communication with the attending physician(s) (for example, rounds meeting)			

Continued on next page

3. Identify methods of admitting cases to the group practice

   v. Establish a method for maintaining information on the group's caseload (for example, a patient roster)

   vi. Establish, prn, a method for exchanging information with ambulatory area

   vii. Other

   i. Identify how admission information will be obtained

   ii. Decide how cases will be admitted to the practice

   iii. Decide how a case manager will be assigned

   iv. Determine the meaning of "length of an episode" for the case type
- When does a "new" case manager assume responsibility?
- How will patient telephone calls be handled (from patient)?
- What type of telephone calls will be made to the patient/by whom?

   v. Other

4. Set quarterly goals relative to the management of the case type

   i. Integrate the case management plan across the episode of illness*

Figure 4-4. (Continued)

Objectives	Activities	Staff	Target Date	Progress Reports
	ii. Complete CMP with physician component/input*			
	iii. Identify case-related learning needs*			
	iv. Other (examples): • Assess targets of opportunity, given the current critical path • Integrate teaching plans/strategies across the episode of illness • Evaluate/improve achievement of specific outcomes • Reduce specific resource utilization			
5. Communicate with attending physician(s)	i. Discuss critical path			
	ii. Introduce concept of case management plan (for later review)			
	iii. Discuss group practice			
	iv. Other			
6. Admit case(s) to group practice	i. Identify potential cases and select case(s) to be admitted			
	ii. Assign a case manager			
	iii. Utilize a critical path and identify variances (record)			

7. Review progress of group practice—*Step I*

    iv. Utilize the case management plan and assess usefulness

    v. Base shift report on critical path

    i. Review variances on critical path; make modifications as needed; identify targets of opportunity

    ii. Review caseload and distributions of assignments; make modifications as needed

    iii. Review systems of communication and make modifications as needed

    iv. Other

Step II

    i. Participate in posttesting

    ii. Review case management plan and make modifications as needed

    iii. Review case management packet and modify as needed

    iv. Review quarterly goals and set new goals

*Initially required goals for all groups.

Source: Copyright, New England Medical Center Hospitals, 1987.

Figure 4-5. Sample Case Management Plan

Diagnosis: __Stroke__   DRG: __14__   MDC: __1__   Length of Stay: __7 weeks__   Unit: __Rehabilitation__

Problem	Outcome (The patient . . .)	Week Visit	Intermediate Goal (The patient . . .)	Week Visit	Process (The nurse . . .)	Week Visit	Process (The physician . . .)	Week Visit
Potential for injury unrelated to treatment (that is, physical trauma)	• Does not experience preventable bodily harm	1	• Verbalizes symptomatology that put him/her at risk for injury	1	• Collaborates with patient/family to establish a safety awareness program appropriate for patient's needs and limitations	1	• Diagnoses cognitive status • Initiates referral to neuropsychologist • Monitors patient's status	1 1 1-7
Risk factors: • Altered mobility • Impaired judgment • Sensory deficits • Lack of skill			• States his/her role and the role of the health care team in the prevention of complications • Complies with preventative measures	2	• Identifies potential complications that necessitate a safety awareness program • Teaches patient activities within patient's safety awareness program • Teaches family the program • Reinforces compliance with the safety awareness program	1 1-7 2-7	• Initiates and follows through on patient/family education and counseling	1-7

Nursing Diagnosis / Etiologies		Expected Outcomes		Interventions	
Disturbance in self-concept/body image		• Accurately describes results of body change and impact on life-style	1–7	• Encourages patient and significant other to talk about diagnosis and its cause	1–2
Etiologies:		• Sets personal goals consistent with physical or functional abilities		• Encourages verbalization of feelings regarding impact on life-style	
• Actual change in structure and/or function or body or body parts		• Verbalizes feelings regarding disability	1–7	• Collaborates with patient to develop a plan of care consistent with patient's needs	1–7
• Nonintegration of change in structure and/or function of body or body parts	1–7	• Actively participates in decisions regarding care		• Elicits patient's opinions and goals for his/her rehab program	1
• Depression		• Identifies support network		• Encourages activities that increase patient's independence	1–7
		• Utilizes identified options for coping with negative feelings		• Focuses on patient's ability rather than disability	1–7
		• Verbalizes strengths	1–7	• Assesses adaptation to disability	1–7
		• Functions at highest level of independence		• Initiates social service and or rehab counseling	1

Continued on next page

Figure 4-5. (Continued)

Problem	Outcome (The patient . . .)	Week Visit	Intermediate Goal (The patient . . .)	Week Visit	Process (The nurse . . .)	Week Visit	Process (The physician . . .)
				1-7	• Assists patient in identifying support network and ways to deal with negative feelings		
				1-7	• Allows time for ventilation of frustration		
				2-7	• Contacts social worker to assist with emotional support, financial concerns, and discharge planning		
Impaired physical mobility *Etiologies:* • Neurological deficit	• Demonstrates a level of mobility that is consistent with assessed functional capacity (specify)	1-7	• Maintains proper body alignment • Does the following (specify with assistance or independently) —Assumes sitting position —Stands —Ambulates —Turns	1-7	• Collaborates with PT team to develop realistic goals, which are reviewed/ revised weekly based on patient's functional ability	1 1 1-7	• Assesses mobility status • Initiates physical therapy consult • Monitors progress both on the unit and with physical therapy

1	• Transfers with assistance	1	• Transfers patient; explains procedure of transfer to patient	• Develops realistic goals based on patient's functional ability
2–4	• Assists nurse with transfer	2–4	• Reviews transfer technique with patient with every transfer • Assists patient in transfer	• Evaluates patient for orthotic equipment
5	• Or significant other demonstrates measures to prevent loss of motion in joints	4–7	• Encourages independent transfer behavior • Ensures ROM is done to affected extremities BID • Teaches and supervises patient with wheelchair propulsion	• Orders any equipment patient requires

Source: Copyright, New England Medical Center Hospitals, 1987.

Figure 4-6. Defining the Nursing Product

- Analyze the patient population
- Focus on high-volume case types
- Identify patient problems by case type
- Identify discharge outcomes
- Establish intermediate goals along a time line
- Relate nursing and physician processes to patient outcomes

Figure 4-7. Potential for Injury/Complication Unrelated to Treatment (Specify diagnosis)

Definition
Presence of risk factors related primarily to the person's general state of health and/or to his or her specific disease symptomatology that could lead to physical injury within the institutional setting (for example, fractures, burns, or head trauma); presence of risk factors that endanger the general health and safety of the patient if appropriate preventive/safety measures are not instituted and/or maintained; presence of a disease or developmental condition, unrelated to treatment, that in and of itself is a contributory causal risk factor for physical injury/harm.

NOTE: This category should only be used if another, specific problem does not address the potential injury—for example, potential for bleeding (as in a hemophiliac).

If there are multiple such potential problems for a single patient, they can be listed as follows:

"Potential for injury unrelated to treatment":
  1. (Specific complications)
     Risk factors
  2. (Specific complications)
     Risk factors

Risk factors
- Altered state of consciousness
- Sensory deficits (visual, tactile, motor, speech, auditory, olfactory, taste)
- Acute reversible confusion
- Environmental conditions [nurse-controlled elements; for example, positioning of bed rails (must be specified)]
- Lack of knowledge
- Lack of skill
- Impaired judgment
- Seizures
- Muscle weakness
- Altered mobility
- Hallucinations
- History of falls
- Stage of physical development
- Stage of psychosocial development

Intermediate goals
- Patient and/or significant other describes the potential symptomatology or complications of this disease state
- Patient and/or significant other states his or her role and the role of the health care team in the prevention of complications
- Patient and/or significant other follows prescribed restrictions or preventive measures (for example, give examples for the case type and/or specify . . . if individual to this patient)
- Patient and/or significant other reports the presence of signs/symptoms of a potential complication
- Patient and/or significant other verbalizes knowledge of safety precautions
- Patient and/or significant other identifies factors that increase potential for injury

Outcome
- Patient does not experience preventable bodily harm

Source: Adapted from Stetler and DeZell (1987).

Figure 4-8. Potential for Complication Related to Treatment (Specify diagnosis)

Definition

Presence of risk factors related to hospital-based treatment of a patient's disease (diagnostic, medical, surgical, procedural, nursing); presence of risk factors, at times inherent in the in-hospital treatment, that endanger the health and safety of the patient if (a) appropriate preventive measures are not instituted and maintained and/or (b) ongoing observation and monitoring are not instituted.

NOTE: This category should only be used if another, specific problem does not address the potential complication; for example, see potential for infection or potential for bleeding.

If there are multiple such potential problems for a single patient, they can be listed as follows:

"Potential for complication related to treatment":
   1. (Specific complication)
      Risk factors
   2. (Specific complication)
      Risk factors

Risk factors

- Administration of medications that have a potential for an adverse or toxic side effect (specify)
- Lack of knowledge (specify)
- Lack of skill (specify)
- Patient noncompliance after appropriate teaching (specify)
- Presence of invasive device or equipment (specify)
- Postoperative status (specify)
- Diagnostic procedures (specify)
- Use of external devices/equipment (specify)

Intermediate goals

- Patient and/or significant other describes the potential complications of the procedure/treatment (for example, give examples for the case type)
- Patient and/or significant other states his or her role and the role of the health care team in the prevention of complications
- Patient and/or significant other follows the prescribed restrictions (for example, give examples for the case type)
- Patient and/or significant other reports the presence of signs/symptoms of a potential complication (for example, give examples for the case type)
- Patient and/or significant other verbalizes knowledge of the prescribed regimen/restrictions
- Patient and/or significant other verbalizes knowledge of reportable signs and symptoms

Outcomes

- Patient does not experience preventable bodily harm
- Patient does not exhibit _____ (state the potential complication and any qualifications)
- Patient exhibits _____ (state the desired patient status)
- Patient reports relief or improvement of expected/anticipated side effects, with appropriate/available treatment (specify)

Source: Adapted from Stetler and DeZell (1987).

Figure 4-9. Potential for Extension of the Disease Process (Specify diagnosis)

Definition
Presence of a specific condition or pathological process that carries with it risks that endanger the recovery of the patient or presence of a risk that will be increased if a treatable extension and/or sequela are undetected.

NOTE: Should only be used if:

a. No other more specific problem addresses the issue
b. Such a problem requires (as a primary intervention) monitoring, observation, and early detection by the nurse
c. Such a problem primarily requires medical intervention or adherence to a medical protocol

Risk factors
- Evolving disease process
- Acute disease process
- Lack of knowledge

Intermediate goals
- Measurements for individual parameters are within the following range (list relevant, critical parameters for the case type)
- Patient and/or significant other reports the presence of critical signs and symptoms
- Patient and/or significant other states his or her role and the role of the health care team in the prevention of disease extension
- Patient and/or significant other verbalizes knowledge of reportable signs and symptoms
- Patient and/or significant other verbalizes knowledge of the prescribed regimen/restrictions
- Patient and/or significant other follows the prescribed restrictions
- Patient and/or significant other verbalizes knowledge of patient's condition, contributing factors and/or potential complications

Outcome
- Patient displays no active symptoms of this complication within our ability to treat (for example, provide examples for the case type)

NOTE: It is recognized that at times no intervention can prevent progression of the disease process; the preceding are therefore the optimum goals for those patients who do respond to treatment.

At times the progression of the disease will change the nature of the patient's status and move him or her into a different case type (and therefore different problems); for example, an uncomplicated MI that becomes a complicated MI.

Source: Adapted from Stetler and DeZell (1987).

Figure 4-10.   Potential for Complication/Self-Care (Specify diagnosis)

Definition

Presence of risk factors that may limit a patient's ability to manage his or her own disease and/or engage in health promoting activities in the "home" environment.

NOTE: If multiple potential problems relative to self-care *at home* exist, then they may be listed as follows:

"Potential for complication/self-care":
1. (Specific complication)
   Risk factors
2. (Specific complication)
   Risk factors

Also note that unlike other categories, other specific potential problems from the standard list may be listed herein as a subheading (for example, infection or injury or bleeding).

Risk factors
- Sensory deficits
- Lack of knowledge (specify)
- Lack of skill (specify)
- Environmental conditions (specify)
- Medication effects
- Impaired judgment
- Ineffective coping
- Language barrier
- History of noncompliance

Intermediate goals
- Patient and/or significant other completes teaching plan
- Patient and/or significant other practices necessary skills (specify)

Outcomes (for inpatients)
- Patient and/or significant other states rationale for prescribed treatments/regimen
- Patient and/or significant other accurately describes . . . (specify the prescribed treatments/regimen)
- Patient and/or significant other accurately demonstrates . . .(specify the prescribed skills for self-care)
- Patient and/or significant other identifies factors that could influence his or her ability to follow the required regimen
- Patient and/or significant other states potential side effects and reportable signs and symptoms

Outcomes (for ambulatory patients)
- Patient does not exhibit signs and symptoms of or experience preventable complication/self-care (specify)
- Patient status is . . . (specify status indicative of absence of the given complication)

Source: Adapted from Stetler and DeZell (1987).

Figure 4-11. Sample Critical Path—Myocardial Infarction

Patient: _____ Case manager: _____ DRG: 122 Physician: _____ Date reviewed: _____ Expected LOS: 6 days

Date	Day 1	Day 2	Day 3	Day 4	Day 5	Day 6	Day 7
Consults	ICU	Cardiac rehab Dietitian	Monitored floor VNA				
Tests	ECG Enzymes	Echo, Muga (if needed)	MBs results: R/I or R/O MI		Holter ETT Cardiac catheterization (if needed)		
Activity	BRP w/ commode		OOB to chair →		Ambulate in room/ hall with assistance →	Up ad lib/ stairs	
Treatments	O₂ Cardiac monitor I&O, weight qd IV		Heparin lock →		D/C O₂ →	D/C (p negative Holter) → D/C (unless CHF) →	D/C →
Diet	No added salt, low-cholesterol diet		Transfer to routine care unit				
Discharge Planning	Assess home environment				Discuss discharge date and needs with MD and family	Discharge orders	Discharge before noon
Teaching	Teaching plans: angina, MI, medication Primary nurse		Discharge class re: medication, risk factors, diet, and smoking				

Admission date: _____ Discharge date: _____ Discharge time: _____ Days in ICU: _____ Days in routine bed: _____

Continued on next page

Figure 4-11. (Continued)

	Variations from Standard		
Date	**Variation**	**Cause**	**Action Taken**

Abbreviations: BRP, bathroom privileges; D/C, discontinue; I&O, intake and output; qd, every day; OOB, out of bed; VNA, Visiting Nurses Association.

Source: Copyright, New England Medical Center Hospitals, 1987.

Financial Implications of Nursing Case Management

An institution's financial health is no longer the sole responsibility of the chief financial officer. Nursing case management integrates clinical goals with financial goals, creating a more unified approach to the business of patient care. This chapter describes the impact of case management on the relationship between financial and clinical outcomes.

□ Management Control versus Operating Control

The relationship between nursing directors and chief financial officers (CFOs) is strained in many hospitals. Nursing represents the hospital's single most expensive department. Nursing salary increases have recently far surpassed hospital price increases. Moreover, the lack of an adequate number of nurses has led many hospitals to close units, which often results in severe financial problems.

The root of the strained relationship is that nursing directors and CFOs often do not think in the same way. Chief financial officers are usually quantitatively oriented. They believe that the essential tool required to manage a hospital is a well-functioning management control system, that is, the planning, budgeting, and monitoring mechanisms that regulate the programmatic and economic activities of the hospital. Nursing, on the other hand, believes that the essential management tool is an operating control system, that is, the mechanisms that ensure the smooth day-to-day functioning of the hospital.

A significant gap exists between the CFO's world of management control and the nursing director's world of operations. This gulf does not appear just in hospitals. Finance and operations are often at odds in other organizations. The conflict, however, seems especially acute in hospitals, particularly in the present difficult economic environment.

☐ Linkage Provided by the Case Management Model

The primary contribution of the case management approach is that it provides a means of linking together the interests of the CFO and the director of nursing. Many efforts have been made in the past in hospitals throughout the country to establish similar linkages. These efforts have largely centered on the implementation of systems that automated nursing functions in a way that helped quantify nursing activities. Examples of these systems include staffing and scheduling, budgeting, and automated nursing care plans.

The problem with most of these systems is that they were designed to measure activity rather than to directly provide cost-effective medical care. Often, these programs have not met the objectives originally promised by their promoters. Because nursing recognized that many of these systems were designed to measure performance, nursing ensured that results were ones that they could support at the operational (patient care) level. In particular, numerous acuity systems have been implemented over the years that are of limited usefulness today because the standards used were developed by nursing departments themselves to explain their own activity.

At New England Medical Center Hospitals, the case management model was not designed to measure, quantify, or play a direct role in the hospital's management control system. Its primary focus was to aid in the operations of the hospital. Despite its lack of financial objectives, however, very significant financial results have been achieved by the nurse case manager. These financial results include significant cost control; lower turnover of nursing personnel; and improved patient satisfaction, which has led to increased occupancy. Each of these issues is discussed in this chapter.

Cost Control

Hospital CFOs largely regard nursing as an expense center, often out of control. A key premise underlying nursing case management is that nursing should be regarded as the activity of the hospital that most directly affects the overall costs of the hospital, not just that of the nursing department.

Since the advent of diagnosis-related groups (DRGs) in 1983, hospital CFOs have learned that the key to cost-effectiveness is not just to reduce intermediate product unit costs such as laboratory, radiology, or nursing costs, but rather to reduce case costs. Countless articles have been written and conferences held about this subject.

It has become widely recognized that clinicians control a significant portion of hospital activities. Most efforts at case management, however, focused initially upon affecting physicians' behavior rather than nurses' behavior. Many of these efforts have been unsuccessful.

Physicians are naturally suspicious of hospital administrators. For most administrators, the primary problem today is to fill empty beds by attracting physicians to use their hospitals, not to control physicians' behavior. Administrators often encounter difficulties in persuading physicians to change their behavior because physicians have different economic incentives than administrators have. Many physicians are still paid on a piecework basis — far different from the case-based payment systems that determine much of hospital revenues.

At New England Medical Center Hospitals, many efforts devoted to improving cost-effectiveness have been initiated by nursing. Physicians have played a strong collaborative role in working with the nurses. However, they have often done so at the request of the nurses rather than the administration. Nursing has played its significant role largely through the development of case management tools (case management plans and critical paths) and systems (group practice models) in collaboration with attending physicians.

Every CFO longs for the day when physicians will agree to prospective normative protocols that call for the use of resources well within payment limits. Unfortunately, it is extremely difficult to get physicians even to admit that such a protocol should be developed, much less to agree on a specific critical path. Nurses have taken on this role and have also taken on the role of involving physicians.

The benefits to nursing of focusing on case management are numerous and well documented elsewhere in this book. From a CFO's point of view, involvement in case management helps to keep the CFO off the nursing director's back. By concentrating on case-oriented cost-effectiveness, nursing has been able to justify more staffing than might otherwise be the case. The cost of an additional few nurses is far less than the benefit of achieving significant reductions in length of stay or ancillary ordering.

Case management provides the linkage between the CFO's management control concerns and the nursing director's operating control concerns. Case management plans and critical paths enable nursing to explicitly describe optimal resource utilization that can be used in developing nursing care plans, the core of nursing operations. The result of this activity, however, is to meet the CFO's need for improved cost-effectiveness.

This is not to say that protocol information regarding optimal paths is not otherwise available to CFOs. Indeed, extensive comparative data bases have been developed to determine how resource utilization differs from hospital to hospital. The problem faced by most administrators, however, is to figure out what to do with comparative information. The dilemma is that cost-effectiveness is impaired in most cases, not because clinicians do not know that fewer resources could be utilized in attaining the same outcome, nor from an unwillingness to provide these fewer resources, but because many hospitals have significant internal constraints that lead to excessive resource utilization. These constraints are intricately built into the operations of the hospital. In many cases, these constraints were themselves designed to achieve cost-effectiveness.

For instance, the radiology department may have developed a methodology of assigning patients within a queue waiting for tests that optimizes the cost of running the radiology department. However, the radiology department does not know that a patient at the end of the queue might be discharged a day or two early if a procedure were done sooner. Optimization of cost is achieved for the radiology department, not for the entire institution.

There are countless rules and procedures governing clinical activity that, in many cases, have been in place for many years and have rarely been examined in terms of their impact on cost-effectiveness. Examples include routine ordering of tests, protocols within intensive care units, and procedures for handling certain types of patients.

Within the framework of case management, cost-effectiveness becomes part of patient care practices. For example, one group practice negotiated for control of four designated beds. In return, they contracted to increase admissions by 10 percent and decrease length of stay by one day for their patients. The group practice accomplished this goal by scheduling all tests prior to admission to cut down on delays. By reducing length of stay, they could admit additional patients on their waiting list. A case manager in hematology talked to the pharmacy department staff about the most appropriate and cost-effective antibiotics for the patient with leukemia.

Case management has been instrumental in identifying hospital operating practices that impede cost-effectiveness. Several group practices set up a series of meetings with a coder from the medical records department to discuss how a specific DRG is assigned and what to document so that their practice is accurately reflected in the assigned DRG. Nurse case managers have worked with the systems department staff to formulate reports that provide weekly, monthly, and quarterly data to help them monitor progress toward goals of cost, length of stay, number of ICU days, delay days, and so forth.

Another example of a dramatic change in practice that affects cost is provided by clinicians engaged in the treatment of ischemic stroke patients. They reported a 29 percent drop in the average length of stay and a 47 percent drop in the average number of ICU days. These patients were able to transfer to rehabilitation services 7 to 10 days sooner. Again, comparative information would not have helped us to resolve these issues. What is needed is for clinicians to look critically at how resources are provided and, in particular, at the institutional constraints that impede cost-effectiveness. It is, then, the process-oriented approach of case management that has been instrumental in helping to improve cost-effectiveness.

The operations of most hospitals still bear the massive effect of 25 years of cost-based reimbursement. Most hospitals have gone through extensive cost-cutting programs primarily oriented toward improving productivity, that is, reducing the quantity of inputs required to provide a test, a procedure, or a patient day of care. Hospital administrators now need to focus on how to change their operations to improve cost-effectiveness.

Nursing is well positioned to play a central role in accomplishing this objective. This is not to say that physicians are not involved but that their involvement is in coordination with nurse case managers. Physicians involved in case management group practices note an increased ability to orchestrate a smooth transition between the different stages of therapy, thus bridging the transition between inpatient and outpatient care. This transition, often difficult, is made easier for the physician as well as for the patient and nurse. Case management programs are ideal vehicles to involve nurses and physicians in helping the hospital improve its level of cost-effectiveness.

Recruitment and Retention

Until a few years ago, CFOs were concerned that there were too many nurses. Today, they are concerned that there are too few. Nursing case management can play a significant role in improving the professional standing and job satisfaction of nurses. This aspect of case management is closely tied to the movement elsewhere in the economy to make work more meaningful.

Until recently, most American managers focused upon what Peter Drucker (1988) has called "command and control" management. Managers have recognized that this traditional approach to organization, emphasizing management control and strong hierarchies, is no longer effective in achieving organizational goals. Instead, strategies that emphasize participative management are seen as far more appropriate. Organizations are adopting the advice of Richard Walton (1987) to move "from control to commitment" as a means of accomplishing objectives effectively. To some extent, this radical change in management reflects a change in the nature of work; to some extent, it is a result of technology that enables individuals to play a far stronger role in directly affecting operations; and to some extent, it reflects the need to recognize that the American work force has changed significantly in the last few years and that individuals demand more autonomy and accountability than in the past.

Case management strengthens the staff nurse's independence and increases the nursing role. As a result, job satisfaction is increased, turnover is reduced, and recruitment is easier. These changes have significant financial benefits. In interviews, nurses note the case management role as one indicator of a progressive and innovative environment in which to practice. The model offers several unique features:

- Being the direct caregiver, a primary nurse is uniquely positioned to best respond to a patient's needs.
- Utilizing a primary nurse as case manager is more cost-effective than introducing another administrative layer to perform this function.
- Offering increased responsibility for clinical decision making enhances the role of the primary nurse, making nursing more rewarding.
- Linking the case manager with the attending physician to coordinate care ensures greater continuity of care throughout the entire episode of illness.

Patient Satisfaction

Most hospitals are actively trying to increase their levels of occupancy. This has proved to be an extremely difficult task because of the overcapacity of hospital beds and increasingly tight utilization control by payers and insurers. As a result, hundreds of millions of dollars are spent by hospitals each year on advertising.

Many hospitals have recognized that, rather than spend millions on televison ads, it would be far more effective to improve their product. Consequently, significant efforts have been devoted to defining outcomes. From a marketing point of view, outcomes are best measured not with sophisticated clinical evaluation but through patient-satisfaction surveys.

Case management has played a significant role in helping achieve patient satisfaction at New England Medical Center

Hospitals. In particular, patients have responded extremely favorably to being told at the outset of their admission (or in some cases, before their admission) exactly how their treatment is expected to take place during their hospital stay. Discussion of critical paths helps patients understand why certain tests are performed and how they relate to overall treatment.

This is not to suggest that hospitals have not discussed treatment plans in the past. They have—through informed consent and the physician's relationship with the patient. However, the primary contribution of nursing case management in achieving patient satisfaction is to enable patients to see the entire episode of illness and to understand how each procedure and activity relates to an overall plan.

As discussed in chapter 4, changes made in treating adult leukemia patients resulted in many benefits and increased patient satisfaction. The length of stay was reduced by more than half, and unnecessary tests were eliminated. The administration of chemotherapy at home eliminated 14 days of hospitalization, resulted in decreases in the infection rate, and allowed patients to spend more time with their families. From such experiences, patients report a feeling of being more in control of what happens to them.

From the CFO's point of view, satisfied patients are one of the hospital's most successful and least costly marketing tools. Patient satisfaction leads to increased occupancy and improves the hospital's financial position.

In summary, the nursing case management program developed at New England Medical Center Hospitals has been instrumental in establishing a link between nursing's concern with operations and finance's concern with profitability. This is not to suggest that in other hospitals CFOs do not care about operations or that nursing directors do not care about costs. However, in most institutions, the framework does not exist to accomplish both goals in a complementary manner. Case management has played a significant role in involving both nurses and doctors in identifying how cost-effectiveness can be improved. Because these programs are initiated by nursing, doctors accept them with less skepticism than they would programs offered by administrators and particularly by CFOs.

☐ Looking to the Future: Automation

Significant work needs to be undertaken in the future to determine how the case management programs can be more integrally related to operation. At this time, case management plans are invaluable sources of information, useful in planning and budgeting. In the future, computerized application of these plans needs to be undertaken to integrate the nursing care plan process with order entry and results reporting. Systems are available on the market and have been implemented in many hospitals that accomplish this objective through a more limited description of nursing care plans. Work needs to be conducted to apply the broader approach of episode-of-illness management to case management plans.

Integration of case management plans within the hospital's patient care system is only the first step of automation. The next step would be to use the critical paths within the case management program to drive the scheduling of services provided within the hospital. Ultimately, this would be performed by optimizing programs that schedule services in order to reduce overall costs of treating episodes of illness rather than to reduce costs of the departments providing services. Finally, case management plans could form the core of an electronic medical record. Ideally, the record would be available to practitioners at multiple sites through terminals. Development of optical scanning technology has led to a number of experimental projects involving this objective.

New England Medical Center Hospitals has been at the fore-front of hospitals in developing automated information systems. It is significant, however, that the case management plans developed at New England Medical Center Hospitals have not been driven by objectives to increase automation. Instead, the focus has largely been on operations and improved cost-effectiveness. The task now is to combine the work on automation with the significant achievements made in controlling costs through managing episodes of illness.

■ *References*

Drucker, P. The coming of the new organization. *Harvard Business Review* 66(1):45, Jan.–Feb. 1988.

Walton, R., and Susman, G. I. People policies for the new machines. *Harvard Business Review* 65(2):88, Mar.–April 1987.

Institutional Implications of Nursing Case Management

We live in a world very different from the one we knew only half a decade ago. The introduction of the diagnosis-related group (DRG) reimbursement system in 1983 radically altered the way hospitals deliver health care. Enormous pressure has been placed upon us to decrease length of stay and discharge patients more quickly to meet DRG pricing guidelines. As a result, patient turn-over is high, and hospitals now primarily care for only the most seriously ill patients. Caring for these patients often requires the services of numerous clinical areas during one stay at the hospital—a predicament that can result in fragmentation of care. All these new challenges on the health care scene have made it clear that the process of patient care needs to be more clearly anticipated, defined, and managed. Only in this way can we balance the demands of cost control and quality of care.

Nursing case management is a promising model for achieving these two goals. The case management plans developed at New England Medical Center Hospitals contain clearly defined goals for optimal length of stay, desired health outcomes, intermediate goals, and processes by which to monitor or achieve these intermediate goals. A nurse case manager, in collaboration with the physician and patient, is responsible for achieving these outcomes within an appropriate length of stay and with effective use of resources. The case manager's responsibilities apply throughout the patient's entire episode of illness, from preadmission, through hospitalization, to discharge.

The case management plan focuses the attention of both nurse and physician upon those aspects of patient care that affect resource utilization, bringing issues of cost containment and operations together for the first time. At New England Medical Center Hospitals, the development of case management plans has often catalyzed a reevaluation of existing protocols and procedures, laying the groundwork for more rational planning and allocation of resources not only on the unit level but also throughout the institution.

This has resulted in dramatic reductions in length of stay and related cost savings. Among the 400–500 myocardial infarction patients admitted to New England Medical Center Hospitals over a two-year period, the average length of stay has been reduced from nine to seven days. During the same period, length of stay for cardiac catheterization patients has been cut from five to two days. Among adult leukemia patients, length of stay has dropped from an average of 49 to approximately 32 days. These are just a few examples of the cost savings that have resulted from the implementation of case management. It must be emphasized that these reductions in length of stay are not affecting quality of care. In virtually all cases, these cost savings are the result of more appropriate care.

It is our belief that fundamental decisions about how to provide efficient high-quality services in this new health care environment cannot be dictated from the top levels of administration down to the clinical units. Nurses and physicians are best equipped to make these decisions about resource allocation. They merely need to be given clear lines of authority and accountability to carry out their decisions. Nursing case management provides an important tool for formalizing these responsibilities.

One of the most compelling arguments for nursing case management is that it allows nurses and physicians to deal generically with the problem of cost-effectiveness on their own terms. They determine the parameters. As a result, a commitment to cost-effectiveness and appropriate utilization of resources is woven into the very fabric of life on the hospital's patient floors and clinical laboratories. The motivation to control costs is instilled and maintained for the most part internally within medical management teams on each floor and through collaborative group practices across a variety of related medical areas.

This approach is much more successful than confronting physicians individually when the cost of cases exceeds DRG payments or conducting detailed studies to determine the cost-effectiveness of care in one hospital relative to care in other hospitals. These approaches tend to elicit defensive responses and do not lead to productive action. Nursing case management has proved to be the most effective approach.

Case management plans place responsibility and accountability squarely where they belong: in nursing. Because nurses are the most knowledgeable about what happens from day to day on the patient units, they are clearly the most logical choice to assume the role of case manager.

At New England Medical Center Hospitals, this accountability is reinforced on numerous levels: (1) in daily informal contact between nurse and attending physician; (2) in weekly meetings of the nursing group practice for specific case types; (3) in monthly consultations on a floor-by-floor basis between nurses and attending physicians to discuss strategic planning of patient care in their discipline; and (4) in quarterly gatherings of senior administrators, physicians, and nurses to identify initiatives that might be taken to further effective utilization of services across related medical areas.

With the case management plan as its guide and reference point, these group meetings provide a helpful forum for the resolution of issues pertaining to operations, resource utilization, and cost control. The formality and clarity of structure are the ingredients of this model's success. Problems not resolved at lower levels inevitably find their way to higher levels. Consequently, a built-in incentive exists for physicians and nurses to address problems in the early stages of identification.

One of the potential strengths of the case management strategy is that, if implemented correctly, it can strengthen the all-important collaboration of nurse and physician. On account of the case management plan, everyone—from the chief executive officer to the staff nurse on the clinical floor—is working from a common vantage point with shared goals and priorities. Channels of communication are opened, enabling nurses and physicians to identify and solve problems efficiently.

This more efficient working environment is a significant asset in recruiting and retaining staff. In today's regulated health care environment, a hospital in which systems and personnel for case management are firmly in place is very attractive to physicians. For nurses, the current staff shortage has only underscored the need to increase job satisfaction. Although salaries must be competitive, it has been proved many times that the most critical elements in job satisfaction among nurses are a sense of independence in decision making, true collaboration with physicians, and respect from physicians and administrators. The nursing case management program accomplishes these goals by giving nurses a sense of participation in the development, monitoring, and management of patient care. The program gives nurses a sense of control over their work through increased accountability and clarification of their role.

One caveat: nursing case management should not be viewed as a way to increase nursing's control over the lives of physicians or managers. If mishandled, the implementation of the case management strategy can become the turf on which territorial battles are fought. Even the term *nursing case management* can be misleading if it limits its institutionwide application.

The nursing case management model is the most effective method devised so far for managing patient care in our present health care environment. The effectiveness of this method depends more than anything else upon collaboration among physicians, nurses, and managers. Therefore, the implementation of this program requires the utmost sensitivity on the part of the nursing staff. Nurses must remain open-minded and capable of resolving conflict through negotiation. No longer can we afford to provide clinical care in isolation. Collaborative conflict resolution is a skill that nurses, doctors, and managers have only begun to develop. Case management is a potential tool for further developing these skills.

One problem chief executive officers (CEOs) may face in establishing nursing case management programs is the potential difference of opinion about the true division of responsibility among doctors, nurses, managers, and even house staff and social workers. In the initial stages of considering the establishment of a nursing case management program, the CEO has to set the stage for success by getting the leadership of these areas to agree that this endeavor is worth undertaking. Interestingly, those at the lower levels usually agree to the idea of a case management strategy; the real barriers to such a plan tend to be in the more senior positions.

Physicians in particular need to be reassured. Time, devotion, and energy must be spent in attempting to get physicians to "buy in to" the program. The following points need to be emphasized:

1. *Physicians still direct overall care,* including making the diagnosis, ordering laboratory tests, prescribing medication, and performing surgery.
2. *Case management plans will not result in "recipe medicine."* The case management plan must be seen as a helpful model, not as a rigid tool. It can and will be adjusted as the physician requires to meet the patient's individual needs.
3. *The case management plan is not a "finger-pointing" tool* but rather a facilitator of internal tracking of a patient's care, with a positive impact on budget planning and resource utilization.
4. *Physicians will reap real benefits from the program.* Prenegotiated systems of care will obviate the need for physicians to completely renegotiate the system of care with each new case. At the same time, quality of care will be maintained.

The CEO can encourage physicians to actively communicate the benefits of the program to fellow physicians, chief residents, and house staff. In this way, positive expectations for the program are developed early at all staff levels.

In conclusion, it must be emphasized that the pressures on resource allocation at the nation's hospitals will not disappear any time in the near future. Thus, senior administrators must begin to actively engage doctors and nurses in the process of containing costs and using hospital resources efficiently. At New England Medical Center Hospitals, nursing case management has proved to be a promising method for accomplishing this goal.

Appendix: Sample Learner Objectives for the Case Management Curriculum

Name _____

Unit _____

Cognitive Domain

___ A. 1. Articulates case management/case manager role in his or her own words.

___   2. Reviews and analyzes case management plans and critical paths that have been produced for the unit's most common DRGs in relation to practicality, comprehensiveness, and so forth.

___ B. Names the basic and expanded management skills necessary to "move" a patient/family from admission to outcome standards.

___ C. Contributes to the nursing staff's knowledge, follow-through, and effectiveness with his or her cases in the following areas:

___   1. Communicates assessments that assist other staff in taking care of the case manager's patient/family.

___   2. Analyzes the way in which each individual patient/family's set of problems evolves over time as more clinical and interpersonal information is gained.

__   3. Determines how outcome standards might be mutually discussed and formulated and interpreted with patients/families. Independently and accurately moves from an interim nursing assessment through the nursing process to a realistic yet comprehensive discharge plan that involves some transition into the community.

__   4. States how intermediate goals can be formulated and revised on a shift-to-shift and day-to-day basis.

__   5. Determines how to organize interventions; communicates them to next shift; utilizes associates and ancillary appropriately.

__   a. Identifies how teaching as an overall healing process facilitates the patient/family's sense of control and self-help capabilities.

__   b. Identifies a potentially difficult situation that would interfere with length of stay or quality care and states what collaborative approaches he or she would use to carry through as a case manager.

__   6. Involves key people on the nursing staff in an analysis of interventions, especially in relation to treatments, and regularly:

__   a. Analyzes the responses of patient/family to teaching over a period of time as more clinical and interpersonal information is gained and clearly communicates this to associates.

__   b. Analyzes case management situations in which collaboration attempts by others were not effective and explains why, using the framework of principled negotiation.

__   c. Analyzes the way in which patient/family's transition into and out of New England Medical Center Hospitals is influenced by case managers.

__   d. Analyzes his or her patterns as a case manager and develops appropriate questions for case management consultation.

Psychomotor Domain

___ A. 1. Independently refers to the case management plans as a standard for practice.

___ 2. Manages own time well.

___ 3. Uses rounds and reports to communicate priority needs from the case management plan or critical paths.

___ B. Attains and sustains relationships with patient/family that demonstrate "professional closeness" in the case manager role.

___ C. Mastery over the nursing process:

___ 1. Constantly uses ongoing, mutual assessments with patients/families to adapt case management plan/critical path.

___ 2. Independently and accurately moves from a nursing assessment to a set of patient problems using the standardized framework.

___ 3. Uses outcome standards as objectives to guide practice. Interprets these to ancillary and professional nursing staff, as well as to patients.

___ 4. Uses intermediate goals to organize the work of other staff. Sets priorities and coordinates activities of self and others.

___ 5. a. Uses problem solving to determine effective interventions; appropriately delegates tasks as necessary.

___ b. Constantly revises and refines patient-teaching to adjust to ongoing assessments of the patient, the health team, and his or her own reactions to the teaching experience. Uses expressive communication techniques (that is, nonjudgmental, open-ended questions) when teaching.

___ c. Calls and conducts a meeting of the health care team as needed.

119

— 6. a. Makes decisions continuously about the case management plan/critical path and communicates these judgments to all staff interacting with patients.

— b. Regularly presents cases for formal consultation from peers.

Affective Domain

— A. Defines accountability in own words.

— B. Discusses opinions about case management with nurse manager and peers.

— C. Nursing process:

— 1. Explains how assessment is integrated into a case manager's daily practice.

— 2. Reads and discusses ideas about nursing diagnoses/patient problems.

— 3. Articulates the value of outcome-based practice.

— 4. Discusses the intermediate goals of other nurses' patients with them.

— 5. Identifies areas of intervention where he or she needs more knowledge or skill, that is, technical, patient teaching, collaboration, and so forth.

— 6. Evaluates self with the case manager checklist. Identifies needs for resources beyond self as they arise.